Upon using the cont
book, you agree to hold
any damages, costs, an.
potentially resulting from the application of any of the information provided by this book. This disclaimer applies to any loss, damages or injury caused by the use and application, whether directly or indirectly, of any advice or information presented, whether for breach of contract, tort, negligence, personal injury, criminal intent, or under any other cause of action.

You agree to accept all risks of using the information presented inside this book.

You agree that by continuing to read this book, where appropriate and/or necessary, you shall consult a professional (including but not limited to your doctor, attorney, or financial advisor or such other advisor as needed) before using any of the suggested remedies, techniques, or information in this book.

Table of Contents

INTRODUCTION

For women who are keen on weight reduction, intermittent fasting may appear to be an extraordinary decision, but numerous individuals need to know, should women fast? Is intermittent fasting effective for women? There have been a couple of key examinations about intermittent fasting, which can reveal some insight into this fascinating new dietary pattern.

Intermittent fasting is also called alternate-day fasting, in spite of the fact there are surely a few variations on this diet. The American Journal of Clinical Nutrition

an examination as of late that enlisted 16 obese men & women into a 10-week program. On the fasting days, participants consumed food to 25% of their assessed energy needs. The rest of the time, they got dietary counselling; however, they were not given a particular rule to follow during this time.

As expected, the members shed pounds because of this study, but what analysts truly discovered fascinating were some particular changes. The subjects were all still plump after only 10 weeks, yet they had shown improvement in cholesterol, LDL-cholesterol, triglycerides, and systolic pulse. What made this an intriguing discovery was that the vast majority needed to lose more weight than these study participants before observing similar changes. It was an interesting revelation that has prodded an extraordinary number of individuals to try fasting.

Intermittent fasting for women has some useful and beneficial effects. What makes it particularly significant for women who are attempting to get in shape is that women have a lot higher fat content in their bodies. When attempting to get more fit, the body essentially consumes sugar stores within the initial 6 hours and afterward begins to consume fat. Women who are following a healthy eating routine and exercise plan might be battling with obstinate fat, but intermittent fasting is a reasonable answer for this.

Intermittent Fasting for Women Over 50

Clearly, women's bodies and digestion change when they hit menopause. Perhaps the greatest change women over 50 experience is they have slower digestion and they begin to put on weight. Intermittent fasting might be a decent method to turn around and forestall this weight gain, however. Studies have demonstrated this fasting design controls hunger and individuals who follow it consistently don't encounter similar longings that others do. In case you are over 50 and attempting to acclimate to your slower digestion, intermittent fasting can assist you with avoiding eating a lot every day.

At the point when you reach 50, your body additionally begins to build up some constants like elevated cholesterol and hypertension. Intermittent fasting has been reported to diminish both cholesterol and pulse, even without a lot of weight reduction. On the off chance you have begun to see your numbers rising at the doctor's office every year, you might have the option to get them down with fasting, even without losing a lot of weight.

Intermittent fasting may not be an extraordinary thought for every woman. Anybody with a particular health condition or who will, in general, be hypoglycemic ought to counsult with a doctor. In any case, this new dietary pattern has explicit advantages for women who naturally store more fat in their bodies and may experience difficulty disposing of these fat stores. There's much more to learn from our subsequent chapters.

Before starting...

Wait a moment! Before getting started I strongly recommend picking up a pencil or a pen; it comes in handy to underline the things that will strike you most or just to jot down the most useful notes, so you don't miss even a chance to learn precious information, thanks to the so-called "*active reading.*"

I read tons of books on dieting and I'm still reading them. The one above is a piece of personal advice that comes directly from my own expertise. It is proven that people manage to *internalize* the concepts they read in any guide when circling the keywords or drawing some lines to link the main concepts... When you *just read* you are more likely to forget things just a few days later. It has also been proved that when you *actively* write - since it involves your active brain functions - you are way more likely to remember things you read and, more importantly, you will surely *act* on them.

So, please. Don't miss this huge chance. That is just a disinterested, yet precious piece of advice.

The 21-Days Intermittent Fasting Journal

During my career as a nutritionist, I've been trying out many tools to help my patients stick to their given plan (some of them are more determined than others, I have to admit it). What I'm going to include in this guide – and you are going to find it right at the end of it - is undoubtedly the most powerful and effective one. And it can help *everyone*.

It consists of a 21-day journal in which you will have to:

- Set your goals and motivation.
- Write down your initial weight and other body measurements into the dedicated progress chart.
- State what you are grateful for during the whole challenge (I do believe in the power of *gratitude*).
- Define your eating window (the hours in which you will respectively eat and fast).

You will also be given other extra space to note down what you are going to do each day, such as working out or food shopping and more.

Why just 21-days?

The answer is easy as pie. It has been scientifically proved that 21 days is the best approximation of the time people need to *master* a habit. If you repeatedly do something for 3 weeks in a row – and this is valid for anything in your life - your mind will adapt to it and it will be a lot easier keep doing it, even for the rest of your life!

But I'm not going to lie to you: it is tough at first. It always was and it forever will be.

Changing habits is hard. But what's good is that once you put in some initial efforts, you will go automatically with your new lifestyle. And the unique tool I created for you makes the whole process a lot simpler to follow.

And on top of that, you will also find some incredibly delicious, yet healthy recipes. They're easy to make and accompanied by simple instructions and useful nutritional values.

Are you ready? Let's get started with this life-changing

guide. Firstly, you will master the theory and finally, you will put everything to practice!

A successful weight loss story by *Anna Sanders*, one of my beloved patients

"I've been discontent with my weight just about all of my life and I've been here and there for whatever length of time that I can remember. Notwithstanding, in September 2014, I had seen an image that was taken of me and my family, and I was completely appalled. I had been experiencing depression, I had pulled back from social situations, and I was hopeless. I felt that it was the point at which I had hit rock bottom and decided I was unable to take it any longer. Around then my weight had gone to a record-breaking peak of 283 pounds. I shunned having pictures taken and missed out on many memories to make with my husband since I was unable to stand seeing myself. I decided the time had come to take care of business."

What caused you to choose to lose weight?

"Numerous things truly! I was seriously depressed and would not take antidepressants. I was unable to inhale, and I could scarcely continue to walk in the shopping center. I was a hopeless, troubled and unhappy person. I needed to be me once more. I wouldn't go anyplace; I wouldn't talk with anybody and I just stayed at home and essentially slept so I wouldn't have to handle the way in which I was feeling. My father has had 3 coronary episodes and coronary illness alongside diabetes, hypertension, and elevated cholesterol all run in my family. I would not like to die due to those health concerns. I didn't care for the person I had become, and I needed to be around to see my girl grow up."

What were the most significant changes you made to lose weight?

"*Most importantly, I needed to re-teach myself how to eat. I likewise needed to finally get it in my head that "intermittent fasting" works. It's a life-changer. It must be something I can do every single day of my life for a mind-blowing remainder. I drink for the most part water and my eating comprises low-fat, low-calorie foods with sensible snacks. I don't place food beyond reach to myself since that makes me need it more.*

If I want a slice of pizza, I will eat it. I simply need to eat less of it, less regularly. Generally speaking, I'm paying special attention to my heart, so I'm taking in less deep fats. What's more, equally as important, I exercise 6 days per week for 60-120 minutes. I exercise at a women's fitness center and I've been there for barely two years. I never figured I could exercise in a rec center before, but since it was all women, I felt increasingly agreeable.

These women were much the same as me and had similar objectives as I did. I do a mix of strength training and heart stimulating exercise through a circuit, with 30 min to an hour on a curved track, and I likewise walk 30 min to an hour outside consistently. In any case, by and large, I would need to state I needed to change the way in which I contemplated getting in shape, exercising and eating right. It's not about looks, it's about my health. I need to be healthy for my children and husband, and I need to teach those qualities to my children so they will carry on with a healthy lifestyle."

What was most challenging about losing weight?

"*Overcoming my fear of exercising particularly around others and learning what to eat, when to eat, and the amount to eat. It sounds simple yet it's a journey. A journey you should be prepared to take. It takes devotion and responsibility. I'm a major passionate eater and I needed to truly dig somewhere within myself and make sense of what started this pattern of passionate eating and why I proceeded with it. When I began managing what was happening inside it was simpler to manage and to lose weight.*"

To what extent did it take you to start to get (see) results?

"*I began getting results within the first two months. The first month I began recording all that I put in my mouth in the Intermittent Fasting Journal you gave me and practiced for 30 minutes per day, 6 days every week. I shed 5 pounds and more than 9 inches.*"

To what extent did it take for you to arrive at your current weight?

"*It has taken me around 2 years to get to the weight I am at now. I accept emphatically that slower is better. Losing it gradually implies you're making the right way of life changes. I haven't taken any diet pills, no unique shots, or anything else. I have done this the ordinary way 100%. I did it by intermittent fasting - changing my dietary patterns and working out.*"

To what extent have you kept up your weight reduction and how do you do it?

"*I'm actually still losing weight at this point. I keep on recording what I eat since I find that encourages me to remain honest. I believe this is a result of the responsibility factor. I additionally still exercise for 6 days every week. I'm extremely dedicated to working out. I know my body needs it, I know my hearts need it, and I know my mind needs it. Exercise is a high for me and it causes me to feel great from head to toe.*"

How has your life changed since you've lost weight?

"*My life has changed to a large extent. I am starting to be me once more. I used to be such an open, bubbly, fun person who was friendly. At the point when I put on all the weight, I withdrew to my home and that was the place I needed to stay. I was discouraged, I would cry, and I was so miserable constantly. Now, I feel astonishing! I'm giggling more, I'm outside more, I accomplish more things with my family, and I'm getting a charge out of being around people once more. I feel the way I used to feel, and I wouldn't change anything for it. I absolutely never need to return to that tragic person I used to be.*"

In what manner will this guide assist the readers with arriving at their weight loss goals?

"*This book will assist and help everyone learn more about weight loss, nutrition, and will provide many fitness tips. It's an amazing inspiration for everybody's journey! I believe information is power, the more you know, the more you learn,*" *and the happier you are. And people will definitely love the information they get from this manuscript!"*

CHAPTER ONE:

WHAT IS FASTING

Intermittent fasting (IF) refers to dietary eating designs that include not eating or seriously limiting calories for a drawn-out timeframe. There is a wide range of subgroups of intermittent fasting each with a particular range in the length of the fast; some for a considerable length of time, others for the day(s). This has become an incredibly well-known subject in the science network because of all of the potential advantages of wellness and health being found.

What is Intermittent fasting (if)?

Fasting or times of intentional restraint from food has been drilled all through the world for a long time, but intermittent fasting with the objective of improving health is moderately new. Intermittent fasting includes confining admission of food for a set timeframe and does exclude any progressions to the real foods you are eating, as of now, the most widely recognized IF conventions are a day by day 16 hour fast and fasting for an entire day, a couple of days of the week.

Intermittent fasting could be viewed as a characteristic eating design that people are driven to follow and it goes right back to our Paleolithic tracker gatherer ancestors. The present model of an arranged program of intermittent fasting might help improve numerous parts of health from body synthesis to lifespan and aging. Despite the fact IF conflicts with the standards of our way of life and basic day by day schedule, the science might be highlighting less eating and more time fasting as the ideal option in contrast to the regular breakfast, lunch, and supper model.

Intermittent fasting is a method that, whenever used appropriately, can enormously improve your health and increase your weight loss. "*Fasting*" is a term used to portray a timeframe when you abandon eating, as is normal in some strict practices. The expression "*Intermittent*" alludes to the range of times for eating and fasting.

Along these lines, intermittent fasting is essentially a training that includes eating inside a specific time and fasting in the time prior and then afterward. We as a whole do this every day since we are not eating when we are sleeping, however, the vast majority of us don't "fast" for long timeframes to get the advantages from it. Let me clarify how you can adjust your method for eating so you can shed pounds very effectively without changing the kinds of foods you eat or the amount of calories you eat.

To take advantage of intermittent fasting, you have to fast for, in any event, 16 hours. At 16 hours or more, a portion of the astounding advantages of intermittent fasting kicks in. A simple method to do this is to just skip breakfast each morning. This is in reality exceptionally sound, yet many people will attempt to disclose to you generally. By skipping breakfast, you are enabling your body to go into a caloric shortage, which will extraordinarily expand the amount of fat you can consume and weight you can lose. Since your body isn't involved with processing the food you ate, it has the opportunity to concentrate on consuming your fat stores for energy and furthermore, for purifying and detoxifying your body.

If you think that it's hard to skip breakfast, you can instead skip supper, even though I find this considerably harder. It truly doesn't make a difference, yet the objective is to expand the timeframe you spend fasting and lessening the amount of time you spend eating. Let's say you have supper at 6 PM, and don't eat until 10 the following morning: you have fasted for 16 hours! Longer is better, however, you can see some quite intense changes from an everyday 16 hour fast.

There are numerous approaches to fasting, and, significantly, you pick what is most appropriate to your way of life so you can stay with it and make it a lifetime propensity. Above, I talked about an everyday fast, however, you can likewise do week after week, month to month or yearly fasts. Every one of them has numerous extraordinary advantages, and I urge you to encounter them for yourself.

Here are two normal myths that relate to Intermittent fasting

Myth 1 - You Must Eat 3 Meals every Day: This "rule," which is normal in Western culture, was not dependent on the proof for improved health; however, it was received as the basic example for pioneers and in the long run turned into the standard. Not exclusively is there an absence of logical basis in the 3-meal a-day model, ongoing studies might be demonstrating not so much meals, but rather more fasting to be ideal for human health.

One investigation indicated that one meal a day with a similar amount of day by day calories is better for weight reduction and body formation than 3 meals every day. This discovery is an essential idea that is extrapolated into intermittent fasting and those deciding to do IF may think that it's best to just eat 1-2 meals every day.

Myth 2 - You Need Breakfast, it's the Most Important Meal of The Day: Many bogus cases about the outright requirement for an everyday breakfast have been made. The most well-known cases being "breakfast builds your digestion" and "breakfast reduces eating later in the day." These cases have been disproved and considered over a multi-week period with results indicating that skipping breakfast didn't reduce digestion and it didn't expand food consumption at lunch and supper. It is as yet conceivable to do Intermittent fasting while still having breakfast, yet some people think it's simpler to have a late breakfast or skip it by and large and this regular myth ought not to disrupt the general flow.

Normal question concerning Intermittent fasting:

Is there any food or drink I am not allowed to eat while Intermittent Fasting? Except if you are doing the altered fasting 5:2 eating regimen (referenced above), try not to eat or drink anything that contains calories. Water, dark espresso, and any foods/drinks that don't contain calories are OK to consume during a fasting period. Truth be told, satisfactory water admission is basic during IF and some say drinking dark espresso while fasting enables a reduction in hunger.

The advantages

The advantages of Intermittent Fasting are immense. Fasting gets negative criticism; however, there is genuine science behind the method of fasting, specifically, Intermittent Fasting. Many people imagine that somebody who is fasting has a dietary issue, yet nothing could be more further from the truth.

In all actuality in the present society, we eat substantially too much and do it over and over again. Our bodies are precise mechanisms that, when allowed to run appropriately, will sustain us a long way past our creative mind. The issue lies with the way that truly, for a great many years, we were a species with little food assets, and we worked long and hard every single day for the amount we got. Today, we have plenty of food, the greater part of it extremely filling, and stationary ways of life. This both adds to obesity and infection.

Fasting Intermittently can wipe out numerous issues caused by indulging and lounging around throughout the day rather than being out hunting and gathering. The truth of the matter is we have not advanced enough to have the option to deal with every one of the calories we ingest consistently, and our bodies still work as though we were hunters and gatherers. Not until the twentieth century did a great many people have food good to go, so 100 years isn't close by anyone's standards to a sufficient opportunity to change how our body works.

Hypertension, elevated cholesterol, and weight are on the whole issues that can benefit from outside intervention with Intermittent Fasting. An especially successful fasting plan is known as the Fast 5. This arrangement expects you to fast for

19 hours every day and eat for 5 back to back hours. Not unreasonably, you DO eat when fasting intermittently. Eating is basic to your health, yet eating a few times per day during a brief period is more normal to our bodies than stuffing them 12 out of 24 hours in a day. Once more, up until the twentieth century, a great many people just figured out how to eat once per day for a huge number of years.

Analysts alert that a couple of solitary studies have been done on people who are exercising intermittent fasts. The impacts of activity and meal recurrence on body formation are fascinating yet to a great extent unexplored zone of research. In any case, there are some positive outcomes. Only a month ago, the *Proceedings of the National Academy of Sciences* distributed a study demonstrating that reducing calories 30% a day expanded the memory capacity of the elderly. In 2007, the journal *Free Radical Biology and Medicine* distributed a study that indicated asthma patients who fasted had fewer manifestations, better brearhing and a decline in the markers of inflammation in the blood than the individuals who didn't fast.

Why is it good for Weight Loss?

Studies show that people who practice Intermittent Fasting can hope to lose up to 7% of their abdomen perimeter, which demonstrates a huge loss of unsafe stomach fat that develops around inner organs and causes sickness. In addition, fasting can decrease insulin resistance, bringing down glucose by 3-6% and insulin levels by 20-31%. It decreases "bad" LDL cholesterol, blood triglycerides, and glucose.

For those of you who have not known about intermittent

fasting, it is the methodology of simply having water and not eating for a time of around 24 hours. For successful fat loss, this ought to be performed 2-3 times each week. Although this may seem like hard work whenever arranged accurately as advanced in *Eat-Stop-Eat*, it is a basic and simple approach to decrease calories while as yet maintaining a full exercise plan. To break down this further we should see fundamental reasons why I think Intermittent Fasting is an amazing arrangement for anyone who needs fast solid weight reduction.

As explained, these fasts are generally completed 2 days per week so as a result, you are reducing just about 2 entire long periods of calorie intake every week. This by itself will promote fast solid weight reduction, as we probably are aware of the premise of all effective weight reduction techniques: devouring fewer calories than you burn off. Be that as it may, if you additionally exercise on these fast days, at that point you significantly increase the amount of fat consumed on those days and consequently speed up the rate which you get in shape. By working out while doing these fasts, you are tackling the issue on two fronts and giving your body no choice to consume fat.

Energy Levels are steady:

A great deal of low-calorie diets and longer fasting type approaches can be exceptionally depleting on your energy levels and do not leave a lot of energy for you to continue working out to a good level. Anyway, with Intermittent Fasting, the inverse has been demonstrated. You regularly have additional energy and faster digestion because of the adrenaline and hormones discharged when fasting for brief periods. This not only enables you to continue working out at a moderate to extreme level yet, in addition, causes a phenomenal fat-consuming condition. On an individual level, I have seen the days that I fast as the absolute most invigorating and gainful days in my week.

Mental and Health Benefits

Apart from the advantage of reducing muscle versus fat levels rapidly, there are likewise other more subtle, yet significant reasons why Intermittent Fasting is a long-haul health path and bad luck for fat. From a health point of view, there is a purification of your body that happens with any fast, as your body acclimates to less food being placed into it.

Also, one that I have seen as extraordinarily helpful is the mental advantages. This is identified by overseeing food, craving, and monitoring all the little triggers that were driving a ton of my eating. Seeing this plainly and improving the control implies you can break the cycle and begin to bring increasingly positive dietary patterns into your life. This is significant for dealing with your weight and health for the present moment as well as for an amazing remainder.

Greatest Fat Loss:

The fundamental motivation behind why you ought to do it is that Intermittent Fasting consumes the most extreme fats. Simply envision, if you fast only for two days every week, you are cutting an entire full two days of calories from your week after week utilization! Also, this, joined with your everyday exercise, can give magnificent outcomes and you will get rid of extra fat.

Keeps up the exercise load quite well:

The second explanation behind fasting is it enables you to keep up a moderate to extraordinary exercise load without losing your energy and digestion, the vast majority of the individuals imagine that fasting channels your energy and digestion, however that is not valid. If you fast in your normal eating routine, you will get more energy and a better capacity to burn calories.

Its Beneficial Aspects:

The third motivation behind why fasting is a decent practice to remember for your exercise plan is its valuable perspectives which give you incredible advantages.

At the point when you do any kind of fasting, your body changes with it by using your muscle versus fat.

It likewise has some mental advantages, similar to you feeling that you are not a prisoner to food.

Intermittent Fasting is the most ideal approach to change your fat burning and exercise schedules. There is no preferred path over Intermittent Fasting of getting the most extreme fat burning by applying a full remaining task at hand.

Obesity Epidemic

As indicated by a huge range of research, the normal resident in America is getting fatter. Since the 1960s, the obesity rate of Americans has quadrupled! It is presently evaluated that at least 25% of American grown-ups are fat, and about 18% of American kids are fat. To figure out how we can start to solve this weight pandemic, keep reading this chapter. All through the article, we will examine why it is essential to turn around the impacts of obesity, just as how we can approach solving this pandemic with a sound, whole foods diet.

How about we start by examining why it is significant that we attempt to explain the obesity epidemic. As the vast majority know, obesity can prompt a wide scope of genuine health confusions. As per questions about it, the obese individuals are at a fundamentally increased danger of developing coronary illness, diabetes, malignant cancers, bone and joint issues, and numerous other real health conditions. It is therefore critical that we start to concentrate on reducing the amount of obesity in the populace, so we can reduce our medical problems and expenses.

Understanding the obesity menace starts with the support of good dieting tendencies. While eating well can once in a while be costly, the settlements are definitely justified despite the expense. We should investigate how eating well can affect our weight and our health.

French fries, pizza, and franks might be scrumptious; however, they will absolutely not assist you effectively with shedding pounds. If you need to get in shape, you need to adhere to an eating regimen that incorporates a wide scope of organic products, vegetables, and whole grains. Every one of these foods will furnish your body with the crucial minerals and supplements it needs to flourish, without harming it with fat, sodium, and calories that cause our bodies to put on weight.

As per research, products of the soil assume a significant role during the time spent for weight reduction and weight on the board. Not exclusively do foods grown from the ground give you minerals, supplements, and nutrients, yet they are likewise low in calories, enabling us to eat enormous amounts without putting on weight.

Products of the soil, in any case, are by all accounts not the only foods that can help in weight reduction measures. Whole grains are additionally significant in weight loss. Whole grain foods contain a lot of fiber, a factor that will keep your body feeling full longer, enabling you to eat less and along these lines consume fewer calories.

As should be obvious, a sound eating routine is the least expensive type of medical coverage you can purchase. Developing smart dieting and an eating regimen loaded with organic products, vegetables, and whole grains is the initial step to understanding the obesity epidemic. To study how a whole foods diet can assist you with combatting weight gain, keep looking through the Web. There are numerous assets out there that can furnish you with nitty-gritty data and good dieting plans that can help you in your own weight reduction objectives.

Pros and cons of Intermittent Fasting

Advancing Health and Weight Loss

Results in a few human studies have discovered that alternate day and whole day Intermittent Fasting has been associated with a noteworthy decrease in body weight, muscle to fat ratio and abdomen periphery both short and long-term, however, has additionally been much of the time seen in some time-limited Intermittent Fasting contemplates.

BRAVO to Increased Brain Functioning!

This is one of the regular advantages of Intermittent Fasting. Studies have investigated the ground-breaking impacts of this time-confined eating routine on subjective execution (for example, memory). If has been seen as advantageous particularly for competitors whether they are exercising or very still (here, here). A 2017 deliberate survey found that weight reduction when all is said in done is related to enhancements in intellectual capacity.

No calorie limitation and No adjustment in diet?

It's hard to believe, but it's true! You can even now eat a similar number of day by day calories and don't need to remove or change the real foods you eat. In any case, we trust you would produce much better outcomes for your health with whole foods, and well-adjusted eating regimens from every one of the 4 food groups.

It's Simple

This eating design is effectively executed and for the individuals who like everyday practice, it tends to be adhered to decently effectively. For certain individuals, it might be anything but difficult to join in your present daily practice. For instance, did you know the normal "Time-confined sustaining" sort of Intermittent Fasting is regularly inadvertently rehearsed by the individuals who skip breakfast and don't have an early supper every day?

Bigger amounts in a shorter timeframe

A few people may like this part a great deal since you find good quick food immediately. This would leave you all the fuller and more fulfilled. As it were, Intermittent Fasting can really keep you from the run of the mill binge of food.

The disadvantages:

Obstruction with the SOCIAL part of Eating

Eating is especially a social action. At the point when you consider it, the all of our festivals, achievements and extraordinary events rotate around food. This new style of eating is totally other from the average every day eating examples of a most people. This is a direct result of the abbreviated time allotment you have for eating. It very well may be hard for you at parties where every other person is eating and drinking, making you fumblingly stand apart from the group.

Also, you may be passing up those late-night sentimental meals, home-made family dinners, birthday meals, lunch gatherings with your chief and associates, and perhaps offering a meal to your mate and children. Not all that good times.

Getting HANGRY, Low in Energy and Unproductive

In a 2016 efficient survey, a couple of researchers found that some Intermittent Fasting members experienced minor unfavorable physical sicknesses including feeling cold, tired, migraines, absence of energy, terrible temper, and absence of focus. We probably won't feel like we have the energy or inspiration to be energetic and do the things we really like!

Devouring = BINGE!

A few people may take the "*Devouring*" periods as a chance to eat a bigger number of calories than they truly need. At the point when you're ravenous, or you foresee a time of fasting coming up, it tends to be enticing to freak out at the main sight of food. If the fasting component in Intermittent Fasting was to make a type of caloric shortage, it's truly conceivable that the eating timeframe effectively fixes it. We should likewise recall that the foods we decide to eat can significantly affect our health. This gorging procedure in the eating routine helps me to remember the It Fits Your Macros diet. This eating regimen centers mostly around how many calories and not the kind of calories. Look at my tirade on the IFYM diet here.

Assimilation Issues

No Difference in Results of Calorie Restriction?

Other examinations have discovered no colossal distinction between consistent calorie limitation and fasting. Huge numbers of the ongoing surveys have not discovered that one procedure is superior to the next, and by the day's end, both yield momentary weight reduction. It is additionally hard to analyze these procedures in view of the distinctive examination techniques and study span. Plainly we need more research, longer-term researches and a bigger example size with a progressively other gathering of members.

Indistinct Impact on Heart

For cardiovascular markers, for example, overall cholesterol, some mixed outcomes were additionally seen in alternate day Intermittent Fasting, in which both LDL (bad cholesterol) and HDL (good cholesterol) increased, while triglyceride levels diminished. Be that as it may, other investigations show that overall cholesterol and LDL diminished (here, here) or HDL continued as before. In an animal study, alternate day fasting reduced overall cholesterol and triglyceride levels. Obviously, we need more human tests on Intermittent Fasting.

Potential Weight GAIN!

Research on Intermittent Fasting's impacts on *metabolism*, there is a diminished dependence on carbohydrates as the fuel source since unsaturated fats are for the most part used in its place. As indicated by researches on momentary fasting, Intermittent Fasting conventions can make glucose fixations decline (decreased glucose oxidation) and lipolysis (unsaturated fat oxidation) to increase essentially during the initial 24 hours. In this manner, Intermittent Fasting can be useful as it advances the breakdown of burning fat.

For what reason should a lady over 50 follow an Intermittent fasting regiment?

No more stressing over food throughout the day - I did the 6 meals per day, cooking all weekend, bundling up dinners to bring with me....and then I asked myself, is this any way to live? That and it wasn't practical or something I would do or appreciate for a mind-blowing remainder, there must be a better method to be healthy.

I can appreciate food when out with companions when I hoose - So I go out and have a few wings and lager on the weekends, generally, I never eat sugar, eat a lot of veggies and meat and just brink water, so the infrequent night out doesn't destroy my "figure" by any means.

It's less expensive - Even despite everything I eat a great deal, I eat less by and large. That and a great many people are typically not cooking at home, so they go purchase their meals. Despite everything I eat 3x per day, it's not tied in with starving myself. Be that as it may, I additionally require fewer calories when I IF, so there are fewer lbs. of meat to purchase. All things considered, I save cash!

No bars or shakes required - Again, I save cash. Every one of the individuals out there pushing you to eat 6x a day are likely individuals who either sell pre-packaged dinners, bars or shakes (ever noticed that?). Try not to misunderstand me, eating 6x a day can work in weight reduction in light of the fact that the day by day all out calorie intske is still low! There's no metabolic bit of leeway to eating 6x versus 3x per day. Eat whole foods 3x per day and make them healthy and you will shed pounds as well! Also, each one of those bars is stacked with sugar, so how does that help insulin resistance?

Increasing mental lucidity and fixation - This is the thing that I notice throughout the day! Astonishing that now only one little Americano in the AM (2 shots expresso in hot water, less caffeine than espresso) will do me fine throughout the day. An explanation for people who have an enormous breakfast or lunch nodding off hours after the fact is because digesting takes a huge amount of energy.

I can gain muscle and lose fat on fewer calories - Again returning to the lifespan of CR here and there, the less you eat the more you will live. Presently despite everything I need to keep my muscle or gain some more now and then. So, I have presently discovered I can do this on IF while requiring way fewer calories than before. Nothing is as sickening as pushing in 5000 calories every day and feeling lazy and tired all to get bigger muscles. Not how I need to carry on with my life.

It feels right - Back in my long stretches of eating throughout the day I felt tired a lot, had expanding joint pain, thought that it was harder to recoup from ice hockey games, had more long periods of despair, and looked and felt fatter. Following a few years of messing with IF I presently feel 1000x better, never again have had knee pain, can recuperate faster from hockey, have shed pounds, have greater lucidity, appreciate life more....and am most likely a lot healthier at 36 than I was at 30! It feels normal to give my body a break from eating to deal with itself, as I don't accept that we were meant to simply live our lives around eating.

Insulin: The way to opening your fat stores

In connection to fat trouble, the key weight reduction hormone is insulin. The less of it you have, the more noteworthy fat you will burn. At the point when your insulin levels are high, the fat in your body won't be consumed as fuel, which is certifiably not a positive result.

Insulin is to some degree like traffic management for your digestion system. Insulin levels keep up hormones, for example, HSL and LPL. HSL is the hormone that pulls the fat from your fat cells with the goal that it will be burned. Ifinsulin is at an elevated level, HSL has no action. LPL resembles the welcome party for your fat cells. It makes proper acquaintance with the new fat. LPL is at a more significant level when insulin is at an elevated level. Insulin has the most movement with regards to refined carbs and natural products. Switch up your beginning of the day bagel for two eggs with cheddar and spinach and it will accelerate your weight reduction process.

Something worth being thankful for about low refined carb eating plans is that you can eat the copy same number of calories and keep on disposing of fat. This implies you could do a little investigation to demonstrate it. Use the details of two health food nuts with a similar weight, sex, and level of activity and put these individuals on 2,000 calorie eating plans. Place one on a low carb diet and the other one on a low-fat eating routine. At the point when the trial is finished, you will find that the individual on the low carb diet will have lost seventy-five to one hundred percent more weight.

This is the principle issue with an eating plan that is loaded up with boring and refined sugars. Fundamentally, the carbs have just two places to go and this is into your muscles/liver as carb stockpiling or into your fat cells. Before they go into your fat cells, they should be changed over into fat first. Your muscle and liver don't have that much space for sugar stockpiling. Nonetheless, sugars are the energy you have to perform a large portion of your day by day exercises. In this way, when you start your day by sitting at your table, in rush hour gridlock, and in your work area seat, you are not using your glycogen stockpile very much. Your muscles and liver are at present completely filled up.

Step by step instructions to improve the Ghrelin levels

Ghrelin is a hormone that makes you feel hungry, however, tests have indicated that this hormone affects your body. An elevated level of ghrelin improves bone composition, restrains insulin discharge, improves endurance rates after a coronary failure, forestalls muscle decay, and may even forestall disease progress and metastasis. In case you're searching for methods to develop ghrelin for a particular health worry, there are a few methodologies you can attempt. For example, adjusting your eating routine and taking supplements. In any case, remember that these procedures probably won't work for everybody. Work with your primary care physician to treat any fundamental conditions and ensure this is a sheltered alternative for you.

Follow a low-fat eating regimen. Eating less fat may increase an expansion in ghrelin. This might be because of the satiety that fat gives. An eating routine that is high in fat decreases ghrelin. By eating less fat, the hormone might be increased. Some low-fat alternatives you may remember for your eating regimen are:

- Low-fat cheddar, milk, and yogurt
- Lean proteins, for example, skinless chicken bosom, ground turkey, egg whites, and beans
- Lower fat versions of foods you typically eat, for example, prepared potato chips, low-fat biscuits, and light bread

Eat twice as high-fiber foods to increase ghrelin in case

you're an overweight or obese postmenopausal lady. Devouring more fiber may increase ghrelin between meals. Eat lots of organic products, vegetables, beans, and whole grains to guarantee that you're getting enough fiber. You may likewise take a daily fiber supplement to advance an expansion in ghrelin.

Aim for 25 grams of fiber every day. In case you're eating almost no fiber presently, build up to this sum over half a month, for example, by adding 1 to 2 servings of high-fiber food into your eating regimen every day.

Use fish oil enhancements to advance ghrelin's mitigating impacts. Omega-3 unsaturated fats raise ghrelin levels. This may have something to do with the calming properties of omega-3s since ghrelin additionally has mitigating properties. Select fish oil supplements or approach your primary care physician for a proposal.

You can likewise get omega-3s from dietary sources, for example, by consuming salmon, mackerel, and pecans.

Get your ghrelin levels verified to see whether they're low. In case you're worried about your ghrelin levels, work with your medicinal services supplier to have them checked and develop a plan for improving them. Your primary care physician can run a blood test to check your ghrelin levels.

- Keep as a top priority that your primary care physician may likewise need to check for other potential reasons for your problem. For instance, in case you're attempting to get thinner, your PCP may likewise check your thyroid.
- Ghrelin levels change and are generally higher around

evening time and lower during the day.

- Western-prepared health providers may not check ghrelin levels since there are no clinical medications or supplements available.

Get treated for conditions that may reduce ghrelin levels. There are a couple of ailments that can cause your ghrelin levels to drop; however, getting treated may increase your levels. Look for restorative treatment on the off chance you have any of the accompanying conditions:

- Polycystic ovary disorder
- Metabolic disorder
- Diabetes type 1 or 2

Lower triglycerides and cholesterol levels

Triglycerides are a sort of unsaturated fat in your body. At the point when you eat a bigger number of calories than you use, your body changes over the overabundance calories into fat as triglycerides and stores it in fat cells. A portion of the triglycerides is continually flowing in your blood. Triglycerides provide an energy hold on your body. At whatever point you need additional energy; your body separates the triglycerides into energy bundles your cells can use.

Abundant triglycerides are flowing in your blood, be that as it may, they can clog your supply routes and cause harm to your pancreas. Ordinary triglyceride levels are beneath 150. If your triglycerides are over 200, they are excessively high. Triglycerides are normally estimated as a major aspect of a "lipid board" that additionally quantifies your cholesterol, including HDL and LDL.

Hazard Factors for High Triglycerides

The most significant hazard factor for high triglycerides is obesity. You are additionally in danger for high triglycerides if you have diabetes, thyroid issues or kidney disease. A few types of high triglycerides are acquired. A few drugs, for example, estrogen, birth control pills, water pills, beta-blockers, and steroids, can cause high triglycerides. Eating a lot of sugar and fat and drinking liquor can likewise cause high triglycerides.

Eating a Healthy Diet to Lower Triglycerides

Diet and exercise are the most ideal approach to bring down your triglycerides. If you can't get your triglyceride levels low enough with diet and exercise, you may need to take triglyceride-bringing down meds. Here are the dietary rules for bringing down triglycerides:

Lower your calories and increase your movement.

You need to use more energy than you take on if you need to bring down your triglycerides. There is no enchantment shot. Sop eating desserts, sugars, and processed carbohydrates. Complex carbohydrates are fine. Complex carbohydrates are found in entire grains, organic products, vegetables, and vegetables. Complex carbohydrates are supplement rich and contain nutrients, minerals, and phytonutrients, including cancer prevention agents.

White sugar is a toxin to you.

It causes your glucose to spike and fall until you create insulin resistance. It contains no supplements, just energy. It changes over very fast to triglycerides. Corn syrup and corn sugars are similarly as awful, and they are in all things. Understand names and watch out for sugars and flavorings. Any fixing that finishes in - one or - ol is most likely some sort of sugar.

Check carbs and don't eat a great deal of fatty, high carbohydrate foods.

Lean meat, leafy foods, and low-fat dairy items should make up the main part of what you eat. Watch the quantity and kind of fat in your eating regimen. Wipe out immersed and Trans fats. Utilize modest quantities of mono-saturated fats, for example, olive oil or canola oil. Include omega-3 fats by eating fish or adding flaxseed to your diet. Try not to drink alcohol. Liquor causes triglyceride levels to rise fast. If you are attempting to bring down your triglycerides, you ought to take liquor out of your eating routine.

Lower cholesterol levels

For a large number of us, when we initially discovered we have elevated cholesterol our first contemplations are to go to cholesterol drug for bringing down cholesterol levels. This is because of the way we regard the assessment of our primary care physicians and statin drugs are normally the principal thing they suggest.

In any case, if you know about the reactions of these prescriptions, at that point, you realize they should just be taken if all else fails. A portion of these symptoms are incredibly serious, including the chance of eternal harm to the kidneys and liver. The same number of up to 25% of people on these medications end up not having the option to tolerate them because of the harm they cause to muscles.

Taking into account how powerful dietary changes are for bringing down elevated cholesterol, it bodes well to find out about the best changes you can make in your eating regimen to bring down cholesterol. The two best things you can do to diminish elevated cholesterol are:

- Reduce the measures of saturated fats in your eating regimen. High-fat meats, for example, hamburger and pork make an interpretation of straightforwardly into more elevated cholesterol and triglyceride levels. Be that as it may, the inverse is additionally valid. By getting rid of these kinds of food from your eating routine, you will rapidly encounter a drop in LDL cholesterol just like your triglyceride readings.
- Increase the amounts of vegetables, organic products, nuts, and whole grains. These are the whole high fiber foods that likewise contain high measures of plant sterols. There is an abundance of logical proof supporting the way fiber wipes out cholesterol from the digestive organs. Simultaneously, plant sterols obstruct the ingestion of cholesterol into the circulatory system.

Bringing down cholesterol levels using this kind of characteristic methodology will really do substantially more than diminish cholesterol readings. Reducing saturated fats and expanding the measures of high supplement foods, for example, these will expel that languid inclination that numerous people with elevated cholesterol experience.

Managing the Symptoms of Menopause

It's not abnormal to hear a great deal of discussion about menopause. Taking into account that each lady more than 50, in the long run, encounters it, it's anything but difficult to perceive any reason why. Menopause is, basically, the discontinuance of the month to month feminine cycle. Essentially, menopause authoritatively signals the finish of a lady's child bearing years.

Past these fundamental logical certainties, however, note that menopause can suffer ruin on a lady's life. By learning the essentials about menopause: what it is, the point at which it happens, what its manifestations are - and how to oversee them - women can get ready themselves and have a greatly improved possibility of traversing this significant life change without hardly lifting a finger.

What Are the Symptoms of Menopause?

By and large side effects of menopause are remarkable. As women approach menopause, they frequently start encountering indications or the like. Truth be told, roughly 70% of women will encounter menopause manifestations. Probably the most widely recognized side effects include:

- Hot flushes
- Night sweats
- State of mind swings
- Weight gain
- Melancholy

For what reason do these indications occur? Hormones are to a great extent at fault. At the point when menopause happens, levels of estrogen and progesterone drop. This decrease in the degrees of hormones can trigger the numerous basic manifestations of menopause.

How do women more than 50 deal with the indications of menopause?

There are a few distinct tips, acts and medications for taking care of and dealing with the indications of menopause. What works for one lady probably won't work for another. One of the most mainstream medicines these days, however, is hormone replacement treatment. Medicinal professionals recommend prescriptions explicit to every lady's requirements.

Certain foods and herbs can likewise have 'estrogen-like' action in the body and can along these lines lessen the side effects of menopause. Eating more soya-based foods, for example, tofu, tempeh, and soya milk, and eating flaxseed meal or oil, will help with manifestations like hot flushes. Herbs, for example, Black Cohosh and Red Clover can be taken in tincture, tea or tablet form and can show an 'estrogen-like' activity too. There are numerous supplements accessible from health food stores and drug stores to help with menopause indications that may contain these herbs.

The following are approaches to deal with the indications of menopause:

- Achieve and Maintain a Healthy Weight
- Intense workout, particularly sex
- Caffeine (espresso, dark tea, colas)
- Drink Enough Water.
- Taking white sugar

- Eat Lots of Fruit and Vegetables
- Spicy food (cayenne, chili beans, ginger, pepper)
- Avoid Trigger Foods
- Eat More Foods That Are High in Phytoestrogens
- Acidic foods (pickles, citrus, tomatoes, capsicum)
- Exercise Regularly

Whatever you experience during menopause, don't leave it unaided as a reason to pass on life. Grasp it and go for it and show the world what an incredible and wonderful lady you are!

CHAPTER TWO

HOW TO FAST

For quite a while, skipping meals was viewed as a terrible method to get more fit. The research demonstrated that skipping meals can slow digestion, which is counter-profitable to weight reduction. Regardless of this, intermittent fasting is a type of abstaining from excessive food intake that is gradually picking up notoriety, particularly among young women, and is by all accounts helping women shed those obstinate, unattractive pounds. It tends to be more earnestly for young women to get thinner than other folks. A promising eating regimen that works and makes it simpler to get thinner is something young women long for.

Intermittent fasting is a kind of diet where the health food nut confines their calorie consumption for at least two days every week. This doesn't imply they don't eat at all on the prohibitive days; they keep their caloric admission to around 500 or 600 calories.

Research presently can't seem to demonstrate why this sort of fasting appears to work, yet results have indicated that all things considered, Intermittent Fasting weight reduction is more noteworthy than weight reduction from consuming fewer calories each day of the week. The straightforwardness of fasting is additionally engaging in light of the fact that individuals don't need to make a decent attempt to eat right.

Intermittent Fasting Plans

Intermittent Fasting isn't simply picking two days to confine calories. There is a real technique to fasting. Here are a couple of the most mainstream strategies:

The 16/8 Method

This Intermittent Fasting plan is when the health food nut doesn't eat for 16 hours out of every day, and at that point eats during a window of 8 hours out of each day. The most straightforward approach to do this is to skip breakfast and not eat at night, yet this is just a recommendation. The window can be set whenever that is agreeable. For more established women, it is proposed to change this technique to 15/9 or even 14/10 since short fasting ranges appear to be better for young women's digestion. The weight watcher can drink something during the fasting time, as long as these ddrinks don't have any calories.

[For a profound understanding of this method, proved to be the most effective one amongst all the other diet protocols, please consider reading the book "Intermittent Fasting 16/8" by Teresa Moore]

The 5/2 Method

This technique includes eating a typical quantity of calories for five days every week and consuming a limited amount of calories two days per week. For young women, it is prescribed to keep their calorie top at 500 during prohibitive days. The days shouldn't be consecutive; they ought to be scattered (for instance, Monday and Thursday).

The Eat-Stop-Eat Method

This technique can be one of the more troublesome strategies. It includes picking two days of the week to quit eating for a whole 24-hour window. The eat-stop-eat technique takes genuine self-restraint. Numerous individuals wind up missing the mark concerning the 24-hour window. Non-caloric drinks are permitted during the 24 hours, so this can make it simpler to finish.

The Warrior Method

The warrior technique is the place the weight watcher only eats an extremely limited quantity of sound, low-calorie foods during the day (leafy foods), and at that point eats a huge supper around evening time. They can just eat one enormous meal. This technique can be marginally hard to follow, however not as troublesome as the eat-stop-eat method.

Intermittent Fasting Can Help Women Lose Weight Fast

Intermittent fasting weight reduction can happen fast when a lady initially starts abstaining from excessive food intake. This is particularly valid for females who are amazingly overweight and have at least 30 pounds to lose. The explanation why this works so well is basic: young women are eating fewer calories when on an Intermittent Fasting plan, the way to guaranteeing that the arrangement works is to not gorge (or under-eat) on days or during windows of customary eating.

Generally, the fasting plans work simply like an eating regimen where you cut calories every day. The greatest distinction with intermittent fasting plans is that these plans make it simpler to cut the calories (regardless of whether they can be difficult to finish, for example, in the eat-stop-eat method). The health food nut doesn't need to forget about calories, make sense of which food is acceptable and which is awful, or make sense of anything so far as that is concerned. They just eat consistently and afterward don't eat. Effortlessness is the thing that makes this eating routine technique successful.

Types of Intermittent Fasting

Regardless of whether you're simply beginning your IF venture or you've taken a stab at fasting previously, but couldn't keep it up long-term, this guide will help. Peruse on to discover the seven unique kinds of fasting and which one is best for your body.

14:10 method

14:10 is a sort of intermittent fasting.

In contrast to the well-known 16:8 method, there is another proportion of fasting and eating periods. Intermittent fasting 14:10 has an eating window of 10 hours and a fasting window of 14 hours. One regular way to deal with doing this is to eat ordinarily in the hours between 9 a.m. and 7 p.m. The period between 7 p.m. and 9 a.m. of the following day is the fasting window.

During the eating timeframe, you can eat your typical dinners and snacks. Moreover, during the fasting window, you are not permitted to eat any calories. Be that as it may, you can drink water and unsweetened espresso or green tea.

Is Intermittent Fasting 14:10 Beneficial?

Any sort of fasting is more rewarding than eating for the duration of the day and night. Accessibility of food and changing way of life has made it feasible for us to eat whenever we need it. This can cause an overabundance of calories, which eventually prompts weight gain.

There are a few advantages of Intermittent Fasting 14:10, for example:

It is simpler to do. If you rest 7 hours every day, doing Intermittent Fasting 14:10 requires just 7 additional long stretches of fasting. This surely looks increasingly feasible, as it has little effect on your everyday calendar and public activity.

Nightly fasting for 13 hours or more decreases the danger of hypertension, elevated cholesterol, and weight gain.

If you need to step up to the 16:8 method or 24hr-fasts, Intermittent Fasting 14:10 can be a phenomenal beginning stage.

Because it has an eating window of 10 hours, you will be more averse to encounter basic reactions, for example, cravings for food, migraines, and expanded fractiousness. Regardless of whether you experience a few, they will be not as serious but rather more workable.

20:4 method

Having an eating window of only four hours is troublesome. So as to go 20 hours without food, you have to work your way up.

It's, for the most part, accepted that the more drawn out the fast, the better. What's more, 20 hours is serious stuff.

A 20:4 split is an extraordinary method to consume the most extra fat.

I will say, however, that getting 1,500 (for instance) calories into only four hours can be a great deal of fun. While you should, in any case, be eating whole, nutritious foods during your eating window, you can bear to be definitely more adaptable than if you were eating a similar number of calories through the span of a whole day. You're still at a caloric shortage so you'll get in shape.

A 20:4 split is the Intermittent Fasting plan I generally return to in light of the fact that it works so well with my life. I don't care for having supper since I don't care for hitting the sack on a full stomach – I like to have an enormous lunch with the goal that I can focus on work.

It additionally doesn't feel like an eating regimen by any means.

At the point when I eat my upkeep calories, I find a workable pace of 1700 calories more than two meals, which is really amazing and keeps me easily full for the whole day. It additionally causes me to hit every one of my macros effectively. It just works for me – and, significantly, you need to locate an Intermittent Fasting plan that works with you as well.

A 20:4 split is regularly alluded to as the Warrior Diet.

In any case, the first 'Warrior Diet', made by Ori Hofmekler 20 years prior is, in reality, all the more a controlled eating routine arrangement than an Intermittent Fasting plan. Ori's Warrior Diet included fasting and eating one primary supper daily, yet nibbling on regular produce outside of that. This is additionally why OMAD is some of the time alluded to as the Warrior Diet too.

The first Warrior Diet was more about the particular foods we eat and bringing down insulin reaction than absolute fasting. The cutting-edge Warrior Diet, be that as it may, will, in general, allude to a 20:4 Intermittent Fasting split.

The warrior method

The warrior diet is an extraordinary type of Intermittent Fasting and is altogether other from the regular three meals per day a great many people are used to.

If you conclude that the warrior diet is something, you need to attempt, slip into the eating routine step by step. Begin by avoiding supper on more than one occasion per week. At the point when you have changed in accordance with that, have a go at stretching out your under-eating periods to the 20 hours required on the Warrior Diet.

What to Eat on the Warrior Diet

When on the Warrior Det, you ought to eat just whole, nutritious, natural foods. What you can eat relies upon which stage you're in.

Serving sizes are not determined and there is no set calorie focus during this eating regimen.

Foods to Eat During the Under-eating Phase

During the under-eating stage, eat just little bits of the accompanying foods:

- Protein: poached or hardboiled eggs
- Dairy: milk, yogurt, curds
- Broth: chicken or meat
- Raw Vegetables: carrots, peppers, mushrooms, greens, onions
- Fruits: bananas, apples, mango, kiwi, peach, pineapple
- Vegetable Juice: beet, carrot, celery
- Small measures of olive oil, apple juice vinegar
- Water, seltzer, espresso, tea
- Foods to Eat During the Overeating Phase
- Protein: chicken, turkey, steak, fish, eggs
- Carbohydrates: potatoes, corn, sweet potatoes, beans
- Grains: pasta, bread, grain, oats, quinoa
- Dairy: milk, cheddar, yogurt
- Cooked Vegetables: zucchini, greens, cauliflower, Brussels sprouts
- Fats: olive oil, nuts

What to Avoid on the Warrior Diet

When following the Warrior Diet, maintain a strategic distance from every single handled food, additives, and food sources with included sugars or sugars.

The accompanying foods are those you ought to stay away from:

- Fast food
- Fried food
- Processed meats like bacon and lunch meat
- Refined sugars
- Candy, treats, cakes
- Chips, saltines

- Canned organic products
- Artificial sugars
- Sweet drinks like organic product juice and pop

The meal skipping

Put down the bagel and read this cautiously: Skipping breakfast could assist you with opening unimaginable medical advantages and live longer. Truly, I'm urging you to break a few dietary guidelines - never skip meals; eat every few hours; breakfast is the most significant meal of the day - that you have been educated since the very first moment. This pattern is "Intermittent Fasting," a dietary convention that in spite of being around for a large number of years is still exceptionally disputable. By moving around your meal times, you actuate certain pathways in your body that could assist you with consuming more fat, secure against specific infections and tumors, and increase your life expectancy - all upheld by logical proof.

Skipping breakfast during IF is well known in light of the fact that you don't see appetite or side effects of fasting while sleeping," says enrolled dietitian Danielle Schaub, culinary and sustenance supervisor for Territory Foods. "It's merely simpler for a great many people to postpone breakfast than it is to hit the hay hungry."

Alright, so perhaps you don't need to skip breakfast to see accomplishments with IF. In any case, will you see more weight reduction, explicitly, when you postpone eating until some other time in the day? This is what specialists state about skipping breakfast when you're doing Intermittent Fasting.

What befalls your body when you skip breakfast?

Unusually, the effect of skipping breakfast on your health and weight is one of the most fervently challenged points in the food world. While the morning meal banter has been continuing for a considerable length of time, more current research recommends that having breakfast doesn't assist you with losing more weight (however skipping it may not, either), as indicated by Harvard Health.

Would you be able to lose more weight when you skip breakfast rather than your other large meals?

Not really. See, if breakfast is your dietary shortcoming, as it were (hi, hotcakes and bacon stacked up with sugary syrup), however, you're regularly increasingly reasonable about lunch and supper, at that point you by and by might see more weight reduction if you skip it. Be that as it may, as a rule, there's no relationship between skipping breakfast and shedding pounds faster. There isn't a convincing exploration that when you eat matters. It's the general calories consumeed in a day compared with whatever number of calories you consume that directs weight reduction.

12:12 method

Essentially, the 12:12 arrangement is a kind of Intermittent Fasting where you eat for 12 hours of the day and fast for the other 12 hours. This method expects you to restrict your day by day calorie admission inside a 12-hour window (which means 12 hours eating, 12 hours fasting), as opposed to eating at whatever point you need for the duration of the day. For example, if you eat your night meal or supper at 8 p.m., you ought to have your morning meal around 8 a.m. the next morning while on this arrangement. The 12:12 is professed to be the least difficult kind of Intermittent Fasting, particularly for tenderfoots who are attempting to get thinner or just need to improve their health.

As per an examination distributed in Cell Metabolism, fasting for 12+ hours most days may advance weight reduction, forestall illness and advance your lifespan. The specialists, who isolated the mice into four eating regimen gatherings and classified them into various sustaining plans, found that mice fasted for at least 12 hours and kept their eating inside a set 12-hour time allotment experienced critical weight reduction contrasted with mice eating a similar eating routine yet with freedom to eat throughout the day.

The analysts likewise found that mice in the time-limited bolstering bunches additionally observed improvements in glucose, insulin, insulin affectability, and craving hormones separated from weight reduction when contrasted with the gatherings of mice who ate at whatever point they needed throughout the day.

Also, other investigations (in the two animals and people) have demonstrated that Intermittent Fasting could be a successful route for getting thinner, particularly gut fat, as it might marginally support your digestion while helping you eat fewer calories. The eating routine arrangement may likewise help digestion and reduce bloating, as well as improve mental lucidity. Probably the best thing about IF is that it might enable the individuals who use it will in general indulge with late-evening eating as fasting can lessen hunger, helping you to adhere to your eating routine arrangement.

In any case, it might be noticed that Intermittent Fasting is unquestionably not for everybody. You should converse with your PCP or health professional before attempting IF, particularly in case you're pregnant or breastfeeding, underweight or living with certain ailments, including diabetes, low blood pressure, and so forth.

5:2 method

Individuals adhering to the 5:2 weight control plans eat standard amounts of healthy foods for 5 days and decrease calorie consumption on the other 2 days. During the 2 fasting days, men, for the most part, devour 600 calories and women 500 calories.

Ordinarily, individuals separate their fasting days in the week. For instance, they may fast on a Monday and Thursday and eat regularly on other days. There ought to be at any rate one non-fasting day between fasting days.

All in all, how does the 5:2 Intermittent Fasting approach work? It's straightforward: You eat regularly 5 days per week and eat just 500 calories (around 25% your ordinary calorie admission) 2 days per week.

Furthermore, what does eating regularly mean? It implies not limiting your calories (utilize my Calorie Calculator if you need assistance making sense of that) and eating whole foods. If you want more rules about what foods to eat, read my Paleo 101 page. It's an incredible beginning stage regardless of whether or not you are anticipating going to Paleo. Normally, individuals don't fast two days straight. What you do is you eat ordinarily three days, fast one day, eat normally 2 days, and fast one day.

Advantages of the 5:2 Intermittent Fasting Diet

The advantages of the 5:2 Intermittent Fasting abstains from food are equivalent to some other kind of Intermittent Fasting technique, which are:

Increases digestion:

We used to stress that any kind of food restriction would hinder our digestion. Remember the guidance to eat like clockwork? Things being what they are, fasting can really build your digestion!

Fights maturing:

The impact of fasting on cell recovery has been very much contemplated. Fasting used on guinea pigs expanded their life expectancy.

Reduces irritation:

Fasting has been seen to diminish inflammation markers (like the C - receptive protein) in your circulation system.

Improves gut health:

Fasting starves off your bad gut microbes, which starve off more rapidly than your good gut microorganisms. I composed an entire post about How Fasting Improves Your Gut Health.

Helps with weight reduction:

It's conspicuous that a general decrease in calories encourages you to get in shape; however, it's more than that. It manages your craving hormones.

What's more, there are a couple of added benefits that are explicit to the 5:2 Intermittent Fasting techniques:

Not stressing over your eating window consistently: I love having more opportunities for the majority of the week. At the point when I practice Intermittent Fasting each day, I sense that I am continually thinking about food and about when I ought to eat.

It keeps your body speculating: The issue with most eating regimens is that your body adjusts and in the long run you hit a weight reduction plateau. This issue can be evaded by switching things up. You are fasting one day, and afterward, you are not fasting. It doesn't hinder your digestion.

Why the 5:2 Intermittent Fasting Diet Works Great for Women

When you have some involvement in fasting, the 5:2 Intermittent Fasting diet is an extraordinary method to accelerate your outcomes without causing hormonal imbalances. Here's the reason:

You can get to your weight reduction objective without continually thinking about food or counting calories: Intermittent Fasting (any method) has been demonstrated to be just as successful as calorie limitation for weight reduction. I had a go at counting calories for half a month. My weight wouldn't move, and I felt unimaginably denied because I was continually confining myself (a shortage of only 500 calories can feel hard to support long-term). Additionally, counting calories for all that you eat can feel dull and tedious. Luckily, there is another way: the 5:2 Intermittent Fasting rearranges calorie checking (read on for the meal ideas) and enables you to live "normally" the remainder of the week.

It is a "sheltered" approach to practice Intermittent Fasting since it doesn't require a day by day fast. We discussed the dangers related to Intermittent Fasting; any method that doesn't expect you to fast day by day guarantees you are not putting a lot of weight on your thyroid and your adrenals.

If you are a lady more than 50 (regardless of whether you are not 50 yet), you will make the most of my post Fasting for Women more than 50, I offer you some accommodating guidance to ensure you benefit as much as possible from your fast as a lady.

5:2 Intermittent Fasting Diet Plan

I referenced as of now that you could use a portion of my fasting plans. Let me share my preferred plans here. They are so natural and delightful!

Apple Almond Salad

- 2 cups chopped apples
- 3 cups chopped lettuce
- 1 cup diced cucumber
- 1 tablespoon flax oil
- 1/4 cup chopped almonds
- Vinegar, salt, and pepper to taste
- Blend everything in a bowl.
- Healthful Information: 512 calories (47% fat, 21% carbs, 16% protein)

Coconut Curry

- 1/4 cup of chopped red onion

- 1 huge red chime pepper
- 1 cup of stripped and chopped butternut squash
- 1 tbsp of coconut oil
- 3 cups of chopped broccoli
- 1/4 cup of tempeh
- 1 cup of canned coconut milk
- Curry powder, and salt to taste

Melt the coconut oil in a pot; include the chime pepper, onion and butternut squash. Cook until the butternut squash is soft. Add the coconut milk, the seasonings, and the broccoli. Cook further until the broccoli is brilliant green.

- Wholesome Information: 514 calories (46% fat, 18% carbs, 42% protein)
- 1/2 tbsp of coconut oil
- 4 cups of mashed cauliflower
- 2 cups of mashed potatoes
- 1 tsp of mashed raw cashews
- Ginger, curry powder, garlic and salt to taste

Melt the coconut oil in a pot, add the potatoes and cook until soft. You may need to include some water with the goal that the potatoes don't stick to the base of your pan. Add the flavoring and the cauliflower and cook until the cauliflower has arrived at the ideal texture.

Does the 5:2 Intermittent Fasting Diet Work for Everyone?

The short answer is nothing works for everybody! As I

referenced above, it's anything but a decent choice for underweight women, have fertility issues or are breastfeeding. If you battle with low blood sugar, feel bleary-eyed or exhausted, you should think about another alternative too. Be that as it may, for a great many people, the 5:2 Intermittent Fasting diet is a fantastic way to deal with getting more fit as well as improving your body and recuperating without following a diet every day. It gives you more slack and enables you to appreciate eating again without continually agonizing over counting calories.

Alternate Day Method

While 5:2 could be viewed as a *"way of life intercession,"* alternative day fasting (ADF) is used to get thinner rapidly. ADF is regularly alluded to as the *"every other day diet"* and expects you to exchange day by day between unhindered eating and devouring an exceptionally low-calorie diet.

Most research on ADF utilizes a comparative way to deal with 5:2, permitting a small meal (for the most part about 500kcal) to be consumed on "fasting" days. Research has demonstrated that ADF can prompt impressive weight reduction in 8-12 weeks, yet a major issue with ADF is that adherence will in general fade away. Longer-term beliefs have indicated that calorie intake on "fasting" days creeps up after some time, which lessens the calorie deficiency accomplished and eases back the pace of weight reduction.

Randomized controlled preliminaries (the highest quality level of clinical research) show that ADF doesn't prompt more weight reduction or enhancements in health compared to traditionally eating less junk food when calorie admission is the equivalent in the two plans. In spite of this, almost certainly, ADF will bring about a more noteworthy decrease in calorie admission compared to customary strategies for eating less junk food, which should prompt more prominent weight reduction, at first. However, it's far-fetched that numerous individuals will cling to ADF in the long-term.

Spontaneous Method

Not into focusing on a particular technique for Intermittent Fasting? You can in any case systematically get some similar advantages by avoiding a meal to a great extent at whatever point you don't feel hungry.

You don't need to follow an organized Intermittent Fasting protocol to receive some of the rewards. Another alternative is to just skip meals every now and then, for example, when you don't feel hungry or are too occupied to even consider cooking and eating.

It's a fantasy that individuals need to eat like clockwork, or they'll hit "starvation mode" or lose muscle. The human body is well prepared to deal with extensive stretches of starvation, not to mention missing a couple of meals every now and then.

In this way, in case you're truly not hungry one day, skip breakfast and simply have a sound lunch and supper. Or then again, in case you're traveling someplace and can't find anything you need to eat, do a short fast. Avoiding a couple of meals when you feel inclined to do so is fundamentally an unconstrained Intermittent Fast.

Crescendo Method

Crescendo fasting and Intermittent Fasting way of life have

helped numerous individuals accomplish their health objectives. Fasting is an old healing system that has been used since the start of known history. Intermittent Fasting is a type of fasting where somebody is fasting 12 to 16 hours or more every day. During this fasting window, you may not be consuming anything aside from water or maybe herbal tea. During the remainder of the day, you would follow a typical, consistent eating regimen.

Intermittent Fasting can have mind-blowing benefits, including lower stress, weight reduction, fat burning, improved energy, better digestion, and improved relationship with food, better mental and profound health, and a lower danger of continual illness.

Be that as it may, male and female bodies respond to fasting in an unexpected way. Women may confront increased difficulties when fasting, including hormonal issues, insulin residence, and affectability to calorie limitation. Notwithstanding, women can even now profit from Intermittent Fasting, however, they may need to alter their methodology. Crescendo Fasting and Cycle Fasting might be amazing Intermittent Fasting systems for some women.

We should jump into finding out about the advantages of Intermittent Fasting, the differences among people more than 50 with regards to fasting, and indications of insulin resistance and diabetes. You will realize why I prescribe a straightforward fast and an early lunch fast to begin with and afterward how to move onto Crescendo Fasting and Cycle Fast safely and effectively. I will likewise go over more than 7 techniques to improve your fasting experience.

Benefits of Crescendo Fasting:

- Being a sensitive approach on a lady's body, this sort of fasting deals with hormonal equalization, which has a significant impact on each lady's life. At the end of the day, your hormones are not thrown into a rage.
- This is a fantastic technique to shed those additional pounds and thin down in an easy wasy.
- The energy levels are likewise kept up to the ideal and in this manner, you probably won't get worn out so easily.

Crescendo Fasting Tips:

- This fasting ought to be done on alternate days during the week, that is to say, for a few days out of every week. As it were, Crescendo fasting ought to be followed during non-consecutive days of the week. For instance, if you eat too much on Tuesday, the following long periods of fasting for you are on Thursday and Saturday.
- Crescendo fasters, in a perfect world fast for around 12 to 16 hours rather than 12 to 20 hours. For instance, if they quit eating at 7 pm, at that point, they don't consume anything till around 9 am the following morning.
- On the days when fasting is attempted, yoga and light cardio activities ought to be one.
- On the days when there is no fasting, exceptional exercises like quality training or Burst/HIIT training ought to be done.
- Do keep yourself hydrated by drinking a lot of water. Refreshments like tea and espresso are fine as long as there is no added milk or sugar in them.

- After about fourteen days, one more day of fasting can be added to the calendar.
- Consider having BCAAs (branched chain amino acids) during your fast days. The quantities being 5-8 grams, branched chain amino acids can renew the protein levels in your body and in this way prevent damage to the muscles. Likewise, it can prevent starvation.
- Crescendo fasting gets its name since you deal with a fasting plan bit by bit that suits your body.

If you experience Intermittent period cycles or certain dietary issues, then perhaps this sort of fasting isn't for you

In light of the remarkable mix of fat burning and medical advantages, Crescendo fasting has gotten exceptionally mainstream, particularly among women.

Rather than oblivious eating, if you follow this kind of fasting to shed those troublesome pounds and remain fit as a fiddle, then we should state that you have embraced a shrewd method for eating and fasting!

Eat-Stop-Eat

At the point when you're on Eat Stop Eat, you take part in obstruction or weight training to keep up and build muscle, as opposed to cardio or other kinds of comprehensive exercise. You don't need to exercise on fasting days; however, you should set up a reliable planning timetable of three to four times each week, with two to four activities for each section, two to five sets for each activity and six to 15 reps for each set.

Eat Stop Eat: Pros

Logical research bolsters Intermittent Fasting as a

compelling weight reduction device. One review, distributed in *Obesity Reviews* in March 2011, found that as long as 12 weeks of intermittent calorie limitation - like the Eat Stop Eat plan - was as successful in weight reduction as reducing calories by a set sum each day; furthermore, it helped health food nuts maintain an increasingly slender bulk. This kind of Intermittent Fasting may deliver other medical advantages as well.

An audit distributed in the journal *Nutrients* in March 2019 found that Intermittent Fasting may improve cardiovascular health by improving blod pressure and cholesterol levels, yet it's not clear if these impacts are because of the weight reduction or the fasting, and clinical investigations are needed.

Pilon refers to decreased stress and cell "purging" as other potential advantages. At long last, Eat Stop Eat might not be so confusing, but rather more direct than counting calories where you need to restrict a whole nutritional category, such as fat or carbs.

Eat Stop Eat: Cons

Fasting each week may not fit your way of life. Richard Bloomer, the head of health sport sciences at the University of Memphis in Tennessee, told the journal CMAJ in 2013, "A great many people won't have the option to do it." Pilon admitted to a similar columnist that Eat Stop Eat is best done secretly because it meddles with normal social collaborations, like meals with family or friends.

The eating routine may cause migraines and grouchiness in certain individuals and is definitely not a reasonable decision for individuals with diabetes, pregnant women or those with a background marked by dietary problems like gorging. The arrangement allows diet beverages, which may actually cause you to long for desserts or pick undesirable foods since you have "saved" calories.

At last, Eat Stop Eat doesn't provide a particular meal plan suggestion for non-fasting days, leaving you to show tremendous poise and decide for yourself what to eat — a territory wherein numerous individuals who battle with their weight need direction.

16:8 technique

16/8 Intermittent Fasting includes constraining utilization of foods and calorie-containing drinks to a set window of eight hours of the day and keeping away from food for the remaining 16 hours.

This cycle can be rehashed as much of the time as you like - from just on more than one occasion for each week to consistently, contingent upon your own inclination.

16/8 Intermittent Fasting has soared in popularity lately, particularly among those hoping to get more fit and burn fat.

While other weight control plans regularly set exacting guidelines, 16/8 Intermittent Dasting is easy to follow and can furnish genuine outcomes with negligible exertion.

It's commonly viewed as not so much prohibitive, but rather more adaptable than numerous other eating routine plans and can without much of a stretch fit into pretty much any way of life.

Notwithstanding upgrading weight reduction, 16/8

Intermittent Fasting is likewise recognized to improve glucose control, help brain capability and improve lifespan.

Many people like to eat between early afternoon and 8 p.m., as this implies, you'll just need to fast medium-term and skip breakfast yet can, in any case, have a reasonable lunch and supper, alongside a couple of snacks for the duration of the day.

Others select to eat between 9 a.m. and 5 p.m., which permits a lot of time for a sensible breakfast around 9 a.m., a typical lunch around early afternoon and a light early supper or snack around 4 p.m. before beginning your fast.

In any case, you can analysis and pick the time allotment that best accommodates your timetable.

Despite when you eat, it's recommended that you eat a few small meals and snacks separated fairly for the duration of the day to help balance out glucose levels and monitor hunger.

Moreover, to expand the potential medical advantages of your eating routine, it's essential to adhere to nutritious whole foods and drinks during your eating periods.

Topping off on supplement rich foods can help balance your eating routine and enable you to receive the benefits that this routine brings to the table.

Take a stab at offsetting every meal with a decent assortment of sensible whole foods, for example,

- Fruits: Apples, bananas, berries, oranges, peaches, pears, and so forth.
- Veggies: Broccoli, cauliflower, cucumbers, leafy greens, tomatoes, and so forth.

- Whole grains: Quinoa, rice, oats, grain, buckwheat, and so forth.
- Healthy fats: Olive oil, avocados, and coconut oil
- Sources of protein: Meat, poultry, fish, vegetables, eggs, nuts, seeds, and so forth.

Drinking no calorie refreshments like water and unsweetened tea and espresso, even while fasting, can likewise help control your hunger while keeping you hydrated. Then again, gorging or trying too hard with lousy food can discredit the constructive outcomes related to 16/8 Intermittent Fasting and may wind up causing more damage than anything else to your health.

[For a profound understanding of this method, proved to be the most effective one amongst all the other diet protocols, please consider reading the book "Intermittent Fasting 16/8" by Teresa Moore]

CHAPTER THREE

FASTING TIPS AND MYTHS

Losing weight is something many women around the world want to do. Intermittent fasting for weight loss is becoming more important. There are many benefits shared and statements made to show how it works. Do intermittent fasting weight loss programs really work? Are they good for your body?

There are also other statements made to show that this type of diet doesn't work; that it's dangerous for you. Are they really right or could you try the diet temporarily?

It's time to work out the truth from the lies. Here's a look at all the myths of Intermittent Fasting to help you find the best weight loss plan for you.

<u>It Is Possible to Lose Weight!</u>

These diets do make it possible to lose weight. There are many myths that state they don't, but studies have shown they do work. This is only when the diets are followed properly.

The benefit is that people can control their hunger pangs. They know that no food is completely off-limit, but that they get to have their meals at a set time. It can also help those who have plans they need to work around or prefer to have strict schedules for their diets.

One of the health benefits noted has been a reduction in insulin resistance. Because there is less glucose from the food, the body doesn't need to release as much insulin during the day. This leads to a lower risk of diabetes.

There are many other health benefits, including hormone regulation and confidence boosts.

It's worth making a note that the diets aren't easy. If losing weight were easy, there wouldn't be any overweight people in the world. This isn't a miracle cure, and you will need to have the motivation to follow the plan.

Why So Many Myths?

If Intermittent Fasting for weight loss is so good, why are there so many myths? Why are people so insistent that this isn't something worth following?

There are many reasons, but the main one is the constant statements; often by people who look like they should know the truths. Bodybuilders will often complain that they're hungry or "experts" may claim that their diet is better for you. Marketers of other diets will say just how bad fasting is for long periods.

The more someone is told something, the more they are likely to believe it. This is especially the case if they are told by people they trust and respect or are told the same thing by multiple people not even in the same friendship group.

Many of the myths are told to promote something else. People will claim one diet is better than the other because they are promoting a specific diet. They don't want to focus on any potential reasons not to try that diet. Celebrities and bodybuilders endorsing certain products for money will also make sure they promote their product and focus on the myths of Intermittent Fasting diets.

There are also mixed results from studies. These mixed results are usually due to limitations in the studies that are taken into account by the people reading the studies. Many will take the studies at face value, rather than comparing how the other studies were carried out and the type of people doing the studies.

This problem has been noted with numerous myths. Researchers have looked into why the studies come out with other results and assess the limitations involved. It could be that people in the studies weren't following a healthy diet plan or that they had medical conditions that affected their ability to lose weight.

It doesn't help that people aren't interested in actually reading through the studies. They don't want to make their own conclusions and will listen to the media or the endorsements instead; often selecting the most damaging or scariest of points to work on their agenda.

You'll Get Fat Skipping Breakfast

Part of Intermittent Fasting involves skipping breakfast. There will be many people telling you this is dangerous and will just make you fat. Breakfast is generally referred as the most important meal of the day.

According to those against Intermittent Fasting weight loss, skipping breakfast will lead to being hungrier throughout the day. Your body already goes through a long fasting period during the night, and it needs food to start your day. If you don't eat breakfast, you're more likely to gorge on food later, and that will lead to weight gain.

The truth is some studies show that skipping breakfast leads to weight gain. There are also studies that show skipping breakfast helps to lose weight.

Those who skip breakfast on a typical day are less likely to be health-conscious with the rest of their meals. They'll snack on high calorie foods. Those who are skipping as part of a weight-loss diet will stick to healthier meals when they do eat.

The main difference in the studies is when they involve children and teenagers. Those who eat breakfast are more likely to do better in school because they find it easier to concentrate.

This is one of those myths that depend on the individual. There are some truths, but if you're following a fasting diet for your weight loss efforts, you will usually find that you lose weight.

Fasting Will Slow Your Metabolism

This is another common myth and can be backed up by those following crash diets. If the body doesn't get enough food, the metabolism slows down to counteract the fewer calories it is getting. Rather than burning the calories your body has stored, it will adapt to survive on less.

It's important to remember that this is an Intermittent Fasting diet. Rather than consuming calories throughout the day, the calories are being consumed in set sittings. There isn't a change to some calories, so there is no need for the body to slow the metabolism down.

Even not getting the full calories for 24 hours won't change much. There are plenty of people who will eat less for 24-48 hours without even meaning to in cases, simply because they don't feel hungry. Their metabolic rates don't decrease because of this. It takes weeks of starvation for the body to go into what is dubbed "starvation mode." Some studies show that it will take 72 hours for the metabolism to drop by just 8%!

You End Up Really Hungry

If you don't continuously eat throughout the day, you'll end up hungry. This is a common belief, and it is time to work out the truth behind it.

Some people may find they feel hungrier by switching from constantly eating to Intermittent Fasting. This is normal because it is a change to the system. However, it really depends on the type of food you eat when you are allowed to eat. If you use your calories up smartly, you can eat food that leaves you feeling fuller for longer, so you don't feel the need to eat as much.

Hunger could also be in the head. People look at the time and think that they need to eat, so they feel hungry. Others will feel hungry because they are thirsty. It can lead to overeating the calories because your body isn't actually crying out for food!

Some people will have a fast snack, but usually not something that will keep them full. Those who do feel the need to snack regularly may find Intermittent Fasting for weight loss much harder. This will come down to the individual, and some will binge later because they have not been able to eat when they've felt hungry. Others will find going hours without food easy, despite the start of feeling hungry.

Smaller Meals Throughout the Day Are Better for You

This myth links to the skipping breakfast and feeling hungry myths. There are believes that eating smaller meals more frequently throughout the day is better for you than eating larger meals at intermittent intervals.

Studies don't show this at all. It all comes back to calories. Eating all your calories in one sitting and eating them spaced throughout the day still means you get the same amount of calories throughout the day. It doesn't change anything about your body! You won't see a reduction in your metabolic rate and your body will still burn the calories.

This will depend on the person, though. It's worth remembering the element about hunger. If you are one of those who really struggle with hunger pangs, then you may find it much harder to have larger meals at intermittent intervals. You may find that eating smaller meals throughout the day is easier for you.

But this is on an individual basis. There's no truth behind the belief that small meals are better for the masses.

Another reason for this myth is the belief health deteriorates without regular food. This is often because people start gorging on unhealthy foods when they feel hungry. Gorging is going to be bad, but sticking to the Intermittent Fasting plan is not going to have an adverse effect. Think about the food that passes your lips and makes healthy choices and you will find your health benefits.

You'll Lose Muscle'

The body goes into starvation mode and then eats at the muscle rather than the stored fats. That's the reasoning behind this myth, but it is not the truth.

It is easy to see where the myth comes from, though. The body can start to eat the calories in the muscles, but that is usually with extreme crash dieting to the point of barely getting any food. It also means the person isn't doing exercise to protect the muscles in the body. As the weight gets so low, the body will start to get the calories from the muscles.

However, for the intermittent plan, the diet isn't going to cause muscle loss. The diet doesn't give your body a chance to do that! You're also still getting plenty of protein to help build the muscle while you lose weight!

Intermittent fFasting is popular with bodybuilders. If it meant a loss of muscle, do you think they'd really still stick to their diets? Wouldn't they move to something that isn't as damaging? The bodybuilders are able to keep their fat percentage low while having the energy to do the workouts they need to build their muscles.

You're not cutting out exercise with this diet. You're not reducing your calories so much that you'll struggle to do it all. You're just getting your calories at strategic points and not as often as you would with a normal eating pattern.

Your Brain Needs the Fuel Constantly

Remember the above about breakfast? Some studies show

children and teenagers work better at school if they have had breakfast. There are a few reasons for this, and those reasons have led to the myth that Intermittent Fasting leads to the brain not getting the fuel it needs. This diet can lead to poor concentration and memory loss.

The truth is that in a developing body it does need the fuel to help. Those children and teenagers who eat breakfast will get the energy they need for their initial start and find it easier to concentrate. Their bodies need extra calories compared to adults, often because they are much more on the go.

When it comes to adults, this is certainly not the case. Some people may find it easier to concentrate, but the brain doesn't just stop working. You won't be at risk of memory problems. If this were true, the human race wouldn't be as big as it is! Just think about the number of people who have gone without food throughout history and have lived, reproduced and helped continue the race.

The belief in this myth is linked to the brain needing glucose (blood sugar). While it does need this, it can also get the energy from proteins. At the same time, the body is very good at regulating everything it needs. It's designed like this, so 24 hours of not eating are not going to affect it negatively! You'll still have the same amount of glucose to keep the brain working.

The biggest reason people believe this is because they focus on hunger. They get it in their head that they can't function properly, and this creates a placebo effect. If they got out of that mindset, they would be able to keep going throughout the day. Like many of the other myths, this is very individually dependent, but science is on the side of the diet.

While the glucose levels within the body will remain stable, there will not be the same response by the body. The pancreas won't release as much insulin, so instead of the myth against the brain, there is the truth that the body benefits from less insulin. There is a lower risk of type 2 diabetes.

The Health Is Negatively Affected

One of the biggest myths told is that health will be affected. You may hear the phrase *"that can't be healthy,"* and it's not because you're not eating that much. It's the type of food you're eating.

There is a belief that those who fast will gorge on food when they are allowed to eat. They'll get all the food that they haven't been allowed throughout the day, and eat too many calories. They'll also make the choice of chocolate over fruity goodness, so they won't get the nutrients the body needs.

However, this isn't the case. Those who are on a specially-designed intermittent diet for their weight loss will make sure they get their nutrients. They will follow a healthy eating plan in the hours they can eat, so they focus on good food that fills them up and gives them energy.

The diets don't cut out water from the diet. People are allowed to drink when they need to, and this can often help to deal with hunger pangs. Their bodies aren't starved of water for hours at a time.

There's No Calorie Deficit

One of the biggest lies out there is you won't create a calorie deficit, but you'll still lose weight. This is a myth that surprisingly a large number of people believe. If this were the case, the diets would be miracle cures, and there wouldn't be anyone overweight!

As mentioned above, diets do create a calorie deficit. They just do it in other ways to normal crash diets or healthy eating plans. For example, the 5:2 diets only creates a deficit over two days. You go back to eating normally for the rest of the week. However, that calorie deficit is a large amount, at around 1,500-2,000 calories each day. This isn't enough to create a starvation mode, though!

The aim of the other five days on this diet is to follow a healthy plan and not overeat the calories. That way the weekly calorie deficit is created to help lose weight one week from the next. If a person has overeaten on calories throughout the week, the fasting won't create the deficit, and there wouldn't be a weight loss at the end of the week.

All Intermittent Fasting diets are like this. They all require a healthy eating plan when someone is allowed to eat. This doesn't just help to create the calorie deficit, but also ensures people get all the nutrients they need throughout the week.

You Won't Lose Weight Because You'll Gain Muscle

This is one of those strange myths that shows people haven't really done their homework. Fat and muscle are two other elements of the body. Neither can change into the other. You can build muscle while you lose fat and muscle can become flabby and look similar to fat, but the fat will not turn into muscle!

The idea you won't lose weight because your body will just turn muscle into fat is ridiculous. Even the idea that you'll lose fat and gain muscle isn't completely true. You will need to do exercise to build and tone muscle. Yes, you can do that on these diets, and you will build some muscle throughout, but it isn't going to replace your fat completely. It takes longer to build the muscle.

The problem is the scales and the way they measure your weight. They take an overall look at your weight, which can take into account fat, muscle, water retention and more without separating them. If you suddenly increase your exercise amounts, it's not going to be a sudden growth of muscle, but your body is countering for the amount of exercise you now do. Follow that plan for a couple of weeks and it will all even out so you go back to losing weight.

A pound of muscle and a pound of fat will be the same. The difference is the amount of space the two take up in the body. Unless you're training for a marathon or fitness competition, there are slim chances you will see the amount of muscle take up the same space as the fat.

You'll Gain the Weight Back Afterwards

When it comes to crash diets, you've likely followed the plan and then just gained it all back again. This is common, and there is a reason for it: you go back to eating the old way. Crash diets don't help you change your habits.

Those who have followed long-term diets will also find sometimes that they gain weight. They get complacent or decide they don't want to stick to the maintenance program for the rest of their lives. It's not the diet that hasn't worked, but their mindset and decisions.

The same applies to Intermittent Fasting weight loss plans. If you don't stick to the maintenance plans, you will end up gaining weight afterward. However, there are maintenance plans because they are lifestyles you can stick to for the rest of your life. This indicates they are healthy and helpful for you.

Those who have found they gained the weight again likely didn't stick to the plan. It may have been a choice they made because they wanted to follow an older plan or it may have been a lack of maintenance. One truth in all this is that maintenance is harder than weight loss because it goes on for much longer. The problem is people would rather blame the plans than their own actions.

The diets do work for the long-term. They are designed to help you lose weight and keep it off in the long run. You just need to have the motivation and determination to succeed at that.

One Plan Didn't Work so the Others Won't Either

There are many other types of Intermittent Fasting plans. Many believe that since one didn't work then, the others won't either. After all, they all have the same idea regarding food and calorie deficits, right?

This is completely wrong. Some diets will be easier for people to stick to while others have elements that people focus too much on that they hate. Having two days where you eat nothing at all may seem too drastic compared to reducing your calories to 500 for two days a week. Likewise, eating only 500 calories for two days may seem too hard for those who would prefer to eat in an eight-hour period seven days a week.

You can only consider yourself and your preferences. Look at your current eating patterns and try the other diets, with the one that sounds most favorable for you first. Weigh them all up against each other and make sure you do put the effort in.

At the same time, you will need to have the determination to succeed. Too many people go into diets believing that they won't work and then find them very hard to stick to. They find any reason for them not to work. If you go in with a negative mindset, you won't find that they do help you lose weight and keep it off afterward.

Should You Follow an Intermittent Fasting Diet?

With all those myths considered, is this something that you should follow for your weight loss? It's not as easy to say yes or no. This really will depend on you as an individual.

Now that you've learned the truth behind the myths, it's up to you whether you believe this is a diet you can stick to. There aren't any tough restrictions on the type of food you can eat, but on the times that you can eat them. You will need to be tough on yourself about sticking to lower amounts of calories on certain days if you're following the likes of the 5:2 diets or sticking to only eating during certain hours of the day.

Overall, you could find that the diets are good for your health. While you reduce the times that you're eating, you're not cutting out nutrients or calories completely. You're just taking them in at other times of the day. It can just get very tempting to snack.

If you need to eat regularly for medical needs (such as taking medication), this is likely not going to be a weight loss plan for you. However, skipping a meal and having your calories later will not affect a normal healthy person. You'd not go to go into starvation mode, and you won't make your brain stop working!

It is a diet worth considering. There are pros and cons to all weight loss programs, but most of the cons of this one are surrounded by myths. Just always remember you should choose the diet that works best for you. The effects may vary, but make sure you don't compromise your health while going through options.

FAQS

How does Intermittent fasting moderate aging?

Scientists note Intermittent Fasting can assist individuals with combatting weight, diabetes, and cardiovascular infection, sicknesses that are hazard factors for age-related illnesses, for example, Alzheimer's. Occasional food limitation brings down cerebrum aggravation and safeguards nerve cells, as shown in animal studies. It additionally initiates autophagy, a cell procedure by which the body stalls and reuses destroyed cell parts. It advances the emission of human growth hormone, which helps you lose weight and raises fat burning.

Would I be able to exercise while fasting?

Research demonstrates that exercising together with IF may reinforce the medical advantages of the two regimens. In a 12-week study using the 5:2 convention (five days of ordinary eating, followed by two days of limited calories), members who followed an activity routine experienced more noteworthy weight reduction than the individuals who just exercised or fasted. A few IF specialists suggest fasting medium-term and exercising toward the beginning of the prior day breakfast. In the wake of fasting medium-term, your muscle's energy stores of glycogen are exhausted. In this way, your body consumes more fat to fuel the work out.

Could Intermittent fasting help with diabetes?

Practically 10% of Americans and Canadians have type 2 diabetes, which might be joined by or lead to other genuine ailments and early death. Mounting research demonstrates that IF may help end the progress of type 2 diabetes. A few specialists recommend that Intermittent Fasting can dispose of the requirement for insulin and manage blood glucose levels. The British Medical Journal distributed a case report in which men fasted - consuming hardly any calories - on alternate days, inside one month of beginning IF, these people weaned themselves off insulin self-injections. After ten months on the IF routine, the men lost a lot of weight and their blood glucose readings fell, and they had the option to decrease their diabetic drugs. Such medications for existing conditions should just be done under the direction of a health professional.

To what extent does it take to become acclimated to Intermittent Fasting?

As per nutrition teacher and fasting scientist Krista Varady, your body may require at least five days to change in accordance with the example of eating and fasting. Specialists recommend novices start with bigger eating windows and steadily extend fasting periods to make the change simpler. They recommend that feeling a little craving is something to be thankful for on the grounds that it helps cultivate a more profound personality body association.

Does it make a difference whether I eat early or late in the day?

Research firmly proposes that the times you eat are as significant as what foods you eat. Because of circadian rhythms, insulin affectability is at its pinnacle early in the day and diminishes as the day advances. Eating later can disturb the circadian beat and elevate the danger of type 2 diabetes after some time. Evening meals will in general trigger more prominent insulin introduction than meals eaten earlier. Huge groups of plausible writing link evening time eating with raised dangers of obesity, cardiovascular illness, diabetes, and even disease. A meta-investigation in the *Annual Review in Nutrition* refers to observational examinations that show caloric admission early in the day may alleviate the danger of these incessant sicknesses.

What would I be able to eat or drink during fasting times?

Intermittent Fasting isn't an eating routine; it's a matter of when you eat or don't eat calorie-bearing foods and beverages. What you consume during your fasting periods relies upon your health objectives. You may decide to remove all foods or refreshments, yet this isn't vital. Whatever IF model you follow, water and other non-caloric beverages are constantly an alternative.

If you choose to consume foods during fasting times, limit your everyday energy intake to 600 calories or less. A little sugar or milk in your espresso once in a while won't harm your fast. Fasting master and creator Dr. Jason Fung urges against diet soft drinks during fasting. Even though they have no calories, the sugar substitutes sway insulin levels and stimulate the craving. Gin Stephens, another fasting master, expresses that protein-rich fluids, for example, a bone stock may obstruct autophagy, which fasting advances.

What do I eat when I'm not fasting?

You can eat and drink whatever you want during your eating period. Food specialists concur that you will profit more from Intermittent Fasting by accepting an eating plan that incorporates whole, negligibly prepared food sources. Foods rich in fiber and protein assist you with feeling full more so you may be happy with less. Reducing refined carbohydrates and oily foods can help lower stress and advance weight reduction. It is significant not to indulge when you end your fasting time, as this could cause stomach pains and damage your health objectives.

How would I manage brain fog or weakness while I'm fasting?

Remain hydrated by drinking a lot of water each day, fasting or not. A few nutritionists maintain that without calories dark espresso can help support energy and fixation. Maintenance systems, for example, meditation may likewise help with brain fog, try low-impact exercise or light physical activity. A few people experience more prominent energy and lucidity with IF.

Do I need to quit eating out with friends to stay with IF?

One of the numerous advantages of Intermittent Fasting is its adaptability. This assists individuals with keeping up their eating and fasting schedules. You can modify your eating plan as per your social plans. If you stray periodically, refocus when you can. While you need to remember your health objectives, you don't need to turn into a slave to them, IF is a direction for living that you can adjust to your own personal calendar. In any case, check with your doctor to ensure Intermittent Fasting is right for you.

CHAPTER FOUR

DELICIOUS AND HEALTHY RECIPES FOR INTERMITTENT FASTING

If you've as of late bounced onto the Intermittent fasting temporary fad, you should be pondering about the foods you can eat. In this subchapter, we'll disseminate a couple of basic Intermittent Fasting recipes you can evaluate whenever you cook. Likewise, we've included Intermittent Fasting veggie-lover plans for those of you who decide to abandon meat!

Intermittent fasting recipes

As it is ordinarily stated, breakfast is the most significant meal of the day. What's more, this is particularly so since it will be the meal you break your fast. Here are some nutritious Intermittent Fasting Breakfast, Lunch, Dinner, Dessert, and Snacks recipes you can evaluate whenever you're in the kitchen.

Breakfast

Chinese-Style Zucchini with Ginger

Nutritional Facts

Servings per container	10
Prep Total	10 min
Serving Size 2/3 cup (55g)	
Amount per serving	
Calories	20
	% Daily Value
Total Fat 8g	6%
Saturated Fat 1g	2%
Trans Fat 0g	-
Cholesterol	0%
Sodium 160mg	9%
Total Carbohydrate 37g	50%
Dietary Fiber 4g	2
Total Sugar 12g	-

Protein 3g	
Vitamin C 2mcg	1%
Calcium 260mg	8%
Iron 8mg	17%
Potassium 235mg	8%

Ingredients

- 1 teaspoon oil
- 1 lb. zucchini cut into 1/4 inch slices
- 1/2 cup vegetarian broth
- 2 teaspoons light soy sauce
- 1 teaspoon dry sherry
- 1 teaspoon roasted sesame oil

Instructions:

- Heat a large wok or heavy skillet over high heat until very hot then add the oil. When the oil is hot, add the zucchini and ginger.
- Stir-fry 1 minute.
- Add the broth, soy sauce, and sherry.
- Stir-fry over high heat until the broth cooks down a bit and the zucchini is crisp-tender.
- Remove from the heat, sprinkle with sesame oil and serve

Breakfast Super Antioxidant Berry Smoothie

Nutritional Facts

Servings per container	5
Prep Total	10 min
Serving Size 4 cup (20g)	
Amount per serving Calories	20
	% Daily Value
Total Fat 2g	5%
Saturated Fat 2g	4%
Trans Fat 7g	-
Cholesterol	2%
Sodium 7mg	9%
Total Carbohydrate 20g	20%
Dietary Fiber 4g	20%
Total Sugar 12g	-
Protein 3g	

Vitamin C 2mcg	15%
Calcium 260mg	7%
Iron 8mg	4%
Potassium 235mg	1%

Ingredients

- 1 cup of filtered water
- 1 whole orange, peeled, de-seeded & cut into chunks
- 2 cups frozen raspberries or blackberries
- 1 Tablespoon goji berries
- 1 1/2 Tablespoons hemp seeds or plant-based protein powder
- 2 cups leafy greens (parsley, spinach, or kale)

Instructions:

- Blend on high until smooth
- Serve and drink immediately

Cucumber Tomato Surprise

Nutritional Facts

Servings per container	5
Prep Total	10 min
Serving Size 2/3 cup (55g)	
Amount per serving Calories	2
	% Daily Value
Total Fat 20g	17%
Saturated Fat 2g	1%
Trans Fat 1.2g	-
Cholesterol	20%
Sodium 55mg	12%
Total Carbohydrate 14g	50%
Dietary Fiber 4g	8%
Total Sugar 2g	-
Protein 7g	

Vitamin C 2mcg	10%
Calcium 20mg	2%
Iron 1mg	5%
Potassium 210mg	7%

Ingredients

- Chopped 1 medium of tomato
- 1 small cucumber peeled in stripes and chopped
- 1 large avocado cut into cubes
- 1 half of a lemon or lime squeezed
- ½ tsp. Himalayan or Real salt
- 1 Teaspoon of original olive oil, MCT or coconut oil

Instructions:

- Mix everything together and enjoy
- This dish tastes even better after sitting for 40 – 60 minutes
- Blend into a soup if desired.

Avocado Nori Rolls

Nutritional Facts

Servings per container	10
Prep Total	10 min
Serving Size 2/3 cup (70g)	
Amount per serving Calories	15
	% Daily Value
Total Fat 2g	10%
Saturated Fat 1g	9%
Trans Fat 10g	-
Cholesterol	1%
Sodium 70mg	5%
Total Carbohydrate 22g	40%
Dietary Fiber 4g	2%
Total Sugar 12g	-
Protein 3g	

Vitamin C 2mcg	2%
Calcium 260mg	7%
Iron 8mg	2%
Potassium 235mg	4%

Ingredients

- 2 sheets of raw or toasted sushi nori
- 1 large Romaine leaf cut in half down the length of the spine
- 2 Teaspoons of spicy miso paste
- 1 avocado, peeled and sliced
- ½ red, yellow or orange bell pepper, julienned
- ½ cucumber, peeled, seeded and julienned
- ½ cup raw sauerkraut
- ½ carrot, beet or zucchini, shredded
- 1 cup alfalfa or favorite green sprouts
- 1 small bowl of water for sealing roll

Instructions:

- Place a sheet of nori on a sushi rolling mat or washcloth, lining it up at the end closest to you.
- Place the Romaine leaf on the edge of the nori with the spine closest to you.
- Spread Spicy Miso Paste on the Romaine
- Line the leaf with all ingredients in descending order, placing sprouts on last
- Roll the Nori sheet away from you tucking the ingredients in with your fingers and seal the roll with

water or Spicy Miso Paste. Slice the roll into 6 or 8 rounds.

MAPLE GINGER PANCAKES

Nutritional Facts

Servings per container	4
Prep Total	10 min
Serving Size 2/3 cup (20g)	
Amount per serving Calories	20
	% Daily Value
Total Facts 10g	10%
Saturated Fat 0g	7%
Trans Fat 2g	-
Cholesterol	3%
Sodium 10mg	2%
Total Carbohydrate 7g	3%
Dietary Fiber 2g	4%
Total Sugar 1g	-
Protein 3g	

Vitamin C 2mcg	10%
Calcium 260mg	20%
Iron 8mg	30%
Potassium 235mg	6%

Ingredients

- 1 or 2 cups flour
- 1 tablespoonful baking powder
- 1/2 tablespoonful kosher salt
- 1/4 tablespoonful ground ginger
- 1/4 tablespoonful pumpkin pie spice
- 1/3 cup maple syrup
- 2/4 cup water
- Mix 1/4 cup + 1 tablespoonful crystallized ginger slices together

Instructions:

- In a neat bowl mix together the first five recipes
- Add flour with syrup with water and stir together, after that add in the chopped ginger & stir until-just-combined.
- Heat your frying pan and coat with a non-stick cooking spray
- Pour in 1/4 cup of the batter and allow it to heat until it forms bubbles. Allow to cook until browned
- Serve warm & topped with a slathering of vegan butter, a splash of maple syrup and garnished with chopped candied ginger.

Chewy Chocolate Chip Cookies

Nutritional Facts

Servings per container	10
Prep Total	10 min
Serving Size 2/3 cup (40g)	
Amount per serving Calories	10
	% Daily Value
Total Fat 10g	2%
Saturated Fat 1g	5%
Trans Fat 0g	-
Cholesterol	15%
Sodium 120mg	8%
Total Carbohydrate 21g	10%
Dietary Fiber 4g	1%
Total Sugar 1g	0%
Protein 6g	

Vitamin C 2mcg	7%
Calcium 210mg	51%
Iron 8mg	1%
Potassium 235mg	10%

Ingredients

- 1 cup vegan butter, softened
- ½ cup white sugar
- ½ cup brown sugar
- ¼ cup dairy-free milk
- 1 teaspoon vanilla
- 2 ¼ cups flour
- ½ teaspoon salt
- 1 teaspoon baking soda
- 12 ounces dairy-free chocolate chips

Instructions:

- Preheat oven to 350°F.
- In a large bowl, mix the butter, white sugar, and brown sugar until light and fluffy. Slowly stir in the dairy-free milk and then add the vanilla to make a creamy mixture.
- In a separate bowl, combine the flour, salt, and baking soda.
- You need to add this dry mixture to the liquid mixture and stir it well. Fold in the chocolate chips.
- Drop a small spoonful of the batter onto non-stick cookie sheets and bake for 9 minutes.

Lunch

Fudge Brownies

Nutritional Facts

Servings per container	9
Prep Total	10 min
Serving Size 2/3 cup (70g)	
Amount per serving Calories	10
	% Daily Value
Total Fat 20g	2%
Saturated Fat 2g	10%
Trans Fat 4g	-
Cholesterol	10%
Sodium 50mg	12%
Total Carbohydrate 7g	20%
Dietary Fiber 4g	7%

Total Sugar 12g	-
Protein 3g	
Vitamin C 2mcg	19%
Calcium 260mg	20%
Iron 8mg	8%
Potassium 235mg	6%

Ingredients

- 2 cups flour
- 2 cups sugar
- ½ cup of cocoa powder
- 1 teaspoon baking powder
- ½ teaspoon salt
- 1 cup vegetable oil
- 1 cup of water
- 1 teaspoon vanilla
- 1 cup dairy-free chocolate chips (optional)
- ½ cup chopped walnuts (optional)

Instructions:

- Preheat oven to 350°F and grease a 9 x 13-inch baking pan.
- Add dry ingredients in a mixing bowl. Whisk together wet ingredients and fold into the dry ingredients.
- If desired, add half the chocolate chips and chopped walnuts to the mix. Pour mixture into the prepared pan and sprinkle with remaining chocolate chips and

walnuts, if using.

- For fudge-like brownies, bake for 20-25 minutes. For cake-like brownies, bake 25-30 minutes. Let the brownies cool slightly before serving.

POMEGRANATE QUINOA PORRIDGE

Nutritional Facts

Servings per container	4
Prep Total	10 min
Serving Size 2/3 cup (40g)	
Amount per serving Calories	22
	% Daily Value
Total Fat 12g	20%
Saturated Fat 2g	4%
Trans Fat 01g	1.22%
Cholesterol	22%
Sodium 170mg	10%
Total Carbohydrate 34g	22%
Dietary Fiber 5g	14%
Total Sugar 7g	-
Protein 3g	

Vitamin C 2mcg	10%
Calcium 260mg	20%
Iron 0mg	40%
Potassium 235mg	6%

Ingredients

- 1 1/2 cup quinoa flakes
- 2 1/2 teaspoons cinnamon
- 1 teaspoon vanilla extract
- 10 organic prunes, pitted and cut into 1/4's
- 1 pomegranate pulp
- 1/4 cup desiccated coconut
- Stewed apples
- Coconut flakes to garnish

Instructions:

- Gently place quinoa & almond milk into a saucepan, & stir on medium to low heat for 9 minutes, until it smooth
- Add cinnamon, desiccated coconut & vanilla extract & taste
- Pit prunes & cut into quarters, add to porridge and stir in well
- Serve in individual bowls
- Add a scoop of stewed apples (kindly view recipe below), pomegranates, prunes & coconut flakes
- Ready to eat!

Stewed apples

- Peel, core, slice apples and place into a saucepan with water
- Cook apples on medium heat, until extremely soft
- Remove from heat, drain & mash apples
- Ready to serve and enjoy your breakfast!

Sweet Corn Soup

Nutritional Facts

Servings per container	4
Prep Total	10 min
Serving Size 2/3 cup (50g)	
Amount per serving Calories	120
	% Daily Value
Total Fat 2g	5%
Saturated Fat 0g	8%
Trans Fat 2g	1.20%
Cholesterol	2%
Sodium 16mg	7%
Total Carbohydrate 7g	10%
Dietary Fiber 4g	10%
Total Sugar 12g	-
Protein 3g	

Vitamin C 2mcg	10%
Calcium 260mg	20%
Iron 20mg	25%
Potassium 235mg	8%

Ingredients

- 6 ears of corn
- 1 tablespoon corn oil
- 1 small onion
- 1/2 cup grated celery root
- 7 cups water or vegetable stock
- Add salt to taste

Instructions:

- Shuck the corn & slice off the kernels
- In a large soup pot put in the oil, onion, celery root, and one cup of water
- Let that mixture stew under low heat until the onion is soft
- Add the corn, salt & remaining water and bring it to a boil
- Cool briefly & then puree in a blender, then wait for it to cool before putting it through a food mill.
- Reheat & add salt with pepper to taste nice.

MEXICAN AVOCADO SALAD

Nutritional Facts

Servings per container	6
Prep Total	10 min
Serving Size 2/3 cup (70g)	
Amount per serving Calories	120
	% Daily Value
Total Fat 8g	10%
Saturated Fat 1g	8%
Trans Fat 0g	21
Cholesterol	22%
Sodium 16mg	7%
Total Carbohydrate 7g	13%
Dietary Fiber 4g	14%
Total Sugar 1g	-
Protein 2g	

Vitamin C 1mcg	1%
Calcium 260mg	20%
Iron 2mg	25%
Potassium 235mg	6%

Ingredients

- 24 cherry tomatoes, quartered
- 2 tablespoons extra-virgin olive oil
- 4 teaspoons red wine vinegar
- 2 teaspoon salt
- ¼ teaspoon freshly ground black pepper
- Gently chopped ½ medium yellow or white onion
- 1 jalapeño, seeded & finely chopped
- 2 tablespoons chopped fresh cilantro
- ¼ medium head iceberg lettuce, cut into ½-inch ribbons
- Chopped 2 ripe Hass avocados, seeded, peeled

Instructions:

- Add tomatoes, oil, vinegar, salt, & pepper in a neat medium bowl. Add onion, jalapeño & cilantro; toss well
- Put lettuce on a platter & top with avocado
- Spoon tomato mixture on top and serve.

CRAZY DELICIOUS RAW PAD THAI

Nutritional Facts

Servings per container	3
Prep Total	10 min
Serving Size 2/3 cup (77g)	
Amount per serving Calories	210
	% Daily Value
Total Fat 3g	10%
Saturated Fat 2g	8%
Trans Fat 7g	-
Cholesterol	0%
Sodium 120mg	7%
Total Carbohydrate 77g	10%
Dietary Fiber 4g	14%
Total Sugar 12g	-
Protein 3g	

Vitamin C 1mcg	20%
Calcium 260mg	20%
Iron 2mg	41%
Potassium 235mg	1%

Ingredients

- 2 large zucchini
- Thinly sliced ¼ red cabbage
- Chopped ¼ cup fresh mint leaves
- Sliced 1 spring onion
- Peeled and sliced ½ avocado
- 10 raw almonds
- 4 tablespoons sesame seeds Dressing
- ¼ cup peanut butter
- 2 tablespoons tahini
- 2 lemons, juiced
- 2 tablespoons tamari / salt-reduced soy sauce and add ½ chopped green chili

Instructions:

- Collect dressing ingredients in a container
- Pop the top on and shake truly well to mix. I like mine pleasant and smooth, however you can include a dash of filtered water if it looks excessively thick.
- Using a mandoline or vegetable peeler, remove one external portion of skin from every zucchini and dispose of.
- Combine zucchini strips, cabbage & dressing in a large

mixing bowl and blend well

- Divide zucchini mix between two plates or bowls
- Top with residual fixings and enjoy it!

KALE AND WILD RICE STIR FLY

Nutritional Facts

Servings per container	3
Prep Total	10 min
Serving Size 2/3 cup (80g)	
Amount per serving Calories	220
	% Daily Value
Total Fat 5g	22%
Saturated Fat 1g	8%
Trans Fat 0g	-
Cholesterol	0%
Sodium 200mg	7%
Total Carbohydrate 12g	2%
Dietary Fiber 1g	14%
Total Sugar 12g	-
Protein 3g	

Vitamin C 2mcg	10%
Calcium 20mg	1%
Iron 2mg	2%
Potassium 235mg	6%

Ingredients

- 1 tablespoonful extra virgin olive oil
- Diced ¼ onion
- 3 carrots, cut into ½ inch slices
- 2 cups assorted mushrooms
- 2 bunch kale, chopped into bite-sized pieces
- 2 tablespoonful lemon juice
- 2 tablespoonful chili flakes, more if desired
- 1 tablespoon Braggs Liquid Aminos
- 2 cups wild rice, cooked

Instructions:

- In a large sauté pan, heat oil over on heater. Include onion & cook until translucent, for 35 to 10 minutes.
- Include carrots & sauté for another 2 minutes. Include mushrooms & cook for 4 minutes. Include kale, lemon juice, chili flakes & Braggs. Cook until kale is slightly wilted.
- Serve over wild rice and enjoy your Lunch!

Dinner

Creamy Avocado Pasta

Nutritional Facts

Servings per container	7
Prep Total	10 min
Serving Size 2/3 cup (25g)	
Amount per serving Calories	19
	% Daily Value
Total Fat 8g	300%
Saturated Fat 1g	40%
Trans Fat 0g	20%
Cholesterol	6%
Sodium 210mg	3%
Total Carbohydrate 22g	400%
Dietary Fiber 4g	1%

Total Sugar 12g	02.20%
Protein 3g	
Vitamin C 2mcg	20%
Calcium 10mg	6%
Iron 4mg	7%
Potassium 25mg	6%

Ingredients

- 340 g / 12 oz. spaghetti
- 2 ripe avocados, halved, seeded & neatly peeled
- 1/2 cup fresh basil leaves
- 3 cloves garlic
- 1/3 cup olive oil
- 2-3 Teaspoons freshly squeezed lemon juice
- Add sea salt & black pepper, to taste
- 1.5 cups cherry tomatoes, halved

Instructions:

1. In a large pot of boiling salted water, cook pasta according to the package. When al dente, drain and set aside.
2. To make the avocado sauce, combine avocados, basil, garlic, oil, and lemon juice in the food processor. Blend on high until smooth. Season with salt and pepper to taste.
3. In a large bowl, combine pasta, avocado sauce, and cherry tomatoes until evenly coated.

4. To serve, top with additional cherry tomatoes, fresh basil, or lemon zest.

5. Best when fresh. Avocado will oxidize over time so store leftovers in a covered container in refrigerator up to one day.

BLACK BEAN VEGAN WRAPS

Nutritional Facts

Sservings per container	5
Prep Total	10 min
Serving Size 2/3 cup (27g)	
Amount per serving Calories	200
	% Daily Value
Total Fat 8g	1%
Saturated Fat 1g	2%
Trans Fat 0g	2%
Cholesterol	2%
Sodium 240mg	7%
Total Carbohydrate 12g	2%
Dietary Fiber 4g	14%
Total Sugar 12g	01.21%
Protein 3g	

Vitamin C 2mcg	2%
Calcium 20mg	1%
Iron 7mg	2%
Potassium 25mg	6%

Ingredients

- 1 1/2 half cups of beans (sprouted & cooked)
- 2 carrots
- 1 or 2 tomatoes
- 2 avocadoes
- 1 cob of corn
- 1 Kale
- 2 or 3 sticks of celery
- 2 persimmons
- 1 Coriander

Dressing:

- 1 Hachiya Persimmon (or half a mango)
- Juice of 1 lemon
- 2 to 3 tablespoons original olive oil
- 1/4 clean cup water
- 1 or 2 teaspoons grated fresh ginger
- 1/2 teaspoon of salt

Instructions:

- Sprout & cook the black beans
- Chop all the ingredients & mix them in a neat bowl with the black beans

- Mix all the ingredients for the dressing & pour into the salad
- Serve a spoonful in a clean lettuce leaf that you can easily roll into a wrap. Most people use iceberg or romaine lettuce.

ZUCCHINI PASTA WITH PESTO SAUCE

Nutritional Facts

Servings per container	5
Prep Total	10 min
Serving Size 2/3 cup (20g)	
Amount per serving	
Calories	100
	% Daily Value
Total Fat 8g	12%
Saturated Fat 1g	2%
Trans Fat 0g	20%
Cholesterol	2%
Sodium 10mg	7%
Total Carbohydrate 7g	2%
Dietary Fiber 2g	14%
Total Sugar 1g	01.20%
Protein 3g	

Vitamin C 2mcg	10%
Calcium 240mg	1%
Iron 2mg	2%
Potassium 25mg	6%

Ingredients

- 1 to 2 medium zucchinis (make noodles with a mandoline or spiralizer)
- 1/2 teaspoon of salt

For Pesto

- Soaked 1/4 cup cashews
- Soaked 1/4 cup pine nuts
- 1/2 cup spinach
- 1/2 cup peas you can make it fresh or frozen one
- 1/4 cup broccoli
- 1/4 cup basil leaves
- 1/2 avocado
- 1 or 2 tablespoons original olive oil
- 2 tablespoons nutritional yeast
- 1/2 teaspoon salt
- Pinch black-pepper

Instructions:

- Place zucchini noodles in a strainer over a clean bowl
- Include 1/2 teaspoon of salt & let it set while preparing the pesto sauce
- Mix all the ingredients for the pesto sauce

- Extract excess water from zucchini noodles & place them in a clean bowl
- Pour the sauce on top & garnish with some basil leaves & pine nuts

BALSAMIC BBQ SEITAN AND TEMPEH RIBS

Nutritional Facts

Servings per container	4
Prep Total	10 min
Serving Size 2/3 cup (56g)	
Amount per serving Calories	100
	% Daily Value
Total Fat 7g	1%
Saturated Fat 1g	2%
Trans Fat 0g	20%
Cholesterol	2%
Sodium 160mg	7%
Total Carbohydrate 37g	2%
Dietary Fiber 2g	1%
Total Sugar 2g	01.20%
Protein 14g	

Vitamin C 1mcg	10%
Calcium 450mg	1%
Iron 2mg	2%
Potassium 35mg	7%

Ingredients

For the spice rub

- 1/4 cup raw turbinado sugar
- 1 or 2 tablespoons this should be smoked paprika
- 1 tablespoon cayenne pepper
- Minced 3 garlic cloves
- 2 tablespoons dried oregano
- 2 tablespoons Kosher salt
- 2 ½ tablespoons ground black pepper
- Minced ¼ cup fresh parsley

Instructions:

- In a clean bowl, mix the ingredients for the spice rub. Blend well & put aside.

- In a small saucepan over medium heat, combine the apple juice vinegar, balsamic vinegar, maple syrup, ketchup, red onion, garlic, and chile. Mix & let stew sit, exposed, for around 60 minutes. Increase the level of the heat to medium-high & cook for 15 additional minutes until the sauce thickens. Mix it frequently. If it appears to be excessively thick, include some water.

- Preheat the oven to 350 degrees. In a clean bowl, mix the

dry ingredients for the seitan & blend well. In a clean bowl, add the wet ingredients. Add the wet ingredients to the dry & blend until simply consolidated. Manipulate the dough gently until everything is combined & the dough feels elastic.

- Grease or shower a preparing dish. Include the dough to the baking dish, smoothing it & stretching it to fit the dish. Cut the dough into 7 to 9 strips & afterward down the middle to make 16 thick ribs.

- Top the dough with the flavor rub & back rub it in a bit. Heat the seitan for 40 minutes to an hour or until the seitan has a strong surface to it. Remove the dish from the heater. Recut the strips & cautiously remove them from the baking dish.

- Increase the oven temperature to about 400 degrees. Slather the ribs with BBQ sauce & lay them on a baking sheet. Set the ribs back in the heater for about 12 minutes so the sauce can get a bit roasted. Then again, you can cook the sauce-covered ribs on a grill or in a grill pan.

GREEN BEAN CASSEROLE

Nutritional Facts

Servings per container	2
Prep Total	10 min
Serving Size 2/3 cup (5g)	
Amount per serving Calories	100
	% Daily Value
Total Fat 10g	12%
Saturated Fat 2g	2%
Trans Fat 4g	20%
Cholesterol	2%
Sodium 70mg	7%
Total Carbohydrate 18g	2%
Dietary Fiber 9g	10%
Total Sugar 16g	01.20%
Protein 2g	

Vitamin C 9mcg	10%
Calcium 720mg	1%
Iron 6mg	2%
Potassium 150mg	6%

Ingredients

- Diced 1 large onion
- 3 tablespoons of original olive oil
- ¼ cup flour
- 2 cups of water
- 1 tablespoons of salt
- ½ tablespoons of garlic powder
- 1 or 2 bags frozen green beans (10 ounces each)
- 1 fried onion

Instructions:

- Preheat oven to 350 degrees.
- Heat original olive oil in a shallow pan. Include onion & stir occasionally while the onions soften and turn translucent. This takes about 15 to 20 minutes, don't rush it because it gives so much flavor! Once the onion is well cooked, include flour & stir well to cook the flour. It will be a dry mixture. Include salt & garlic powder. Add some water. Let simmer for about 1 – 2 minutes & allow the mixture to thicken. Immediately remove from heat.
- Pour green beans into a square baking dish & add 2/3 can of onions. Include all of the gravy & stir well to together.

- Place in oven & cook for 25 to 30 minutes, gravy mixture will be bubbly. Top with remaining fried onions & cook for 4 to 12 minutes more. Serve immediately and enjoy your dinner.

SOCCA PIZZA [VEGAN]

Nutritional Facts

Servings per container	2
Prep Total	10 min
Serving Size 2/3 cup (78g)	
Amount per serving Calories	120
	% Daily Value
Total Fat 10g	20%
Saturated Fat 5g	7%
Trans Fat 6g	27%
Cholesterol	5%
Sodium 10mg	10%
Total Carbohydrate 4g	20%
Dietary Fiber 9g	15%
Total Sugar 12g	01.70%
Protein 6g	

Vitamin C 7mcg	10%
Calcium 290mg	20%
Iron 4mg	2%
Potassium 240mg	7%

Ingredients

Socca Base

- 1 cup chickpea (garbanzo bean) flour – I used-Bob's Red Mill Garbanzo Fava Flour
- 1 or 2 cups of cold, filtered water
- 1 to 2 tablespoons of minced garlic
- ½ tablespoon of sea salt
- 2 tablespoons of coconut oil (for greasing)

Toppings

- Add Tomato-paste
- Add Dried Italian herbs (oregano, basil, thyme, rosemary, etc.)
- Add Mushrooms
- Add Red onion
- Add Capsicum/bell pepper
- Add Sun-dried tomatoes
- Add Kalamata olives
- Add Vegan Cheese & Chopped Fresh basil leaves

Instructions:

- Pre-heat oven to 350F.
- In a clean mixing bowl, whisk together garbanzo bean

flour & water until there are no lumps remaining. Stir together in garlic and sea salt. Allow to rest for about 12 minutes to thicken.

- Grease 2 - 4 small, shallow dishes/tins with original coconut oil.
- Pour mixture into a clean dish & bake for about 20 - 15 minutes or until golden brown.
- Remove dishes from the oven, top with your favorite toppings & vegan cheese (optional) & return to the oven for another 7 - 10 minutes or so.
- Remove dishes from oven & allow to sit for about 2 – 5 minutes before removing pizzas from the dishes. Enjoy your dinner!

Dessert & snacks

VEGAN SNAKE RECIPES

I t is mid-morning and you're feeling a little peckish - what will you eat? You feel a bit deprived because you are on the vegan diet, and you can't think of any tasty and fast snack ideas. Or perhaps you've just come home from work and are craving a yummy treat, but you are tired. You, therefore, want your vegan snack to be easy, hassle-free, and not one of the most complicated time-consuming recipes on the planet, even better - preferably just something that you can throw together in under 5 or 10 minutes.

Below is a list of some tasty, fast and easy vegan snacks recipes and food ideas to help make your life a little easier.

Popcorn

It's a tasty, rather low-calorie snack that can be ready to eat in under 10 minutes. It's perfect if you're craving something a little salty.

Nutritional Facts

Servings per container	5
Prep Total	10 min

Serving Size	8
Amount per serving Calories	0%
	% Daily Value
Total Fat 3g	20%
Saturated Fat 4g	32%
Trans Fat 2g	2%
Cholesterol	2%
Sodium 110mg	0.2%
Total Carbohydrate 21g	50%
Dietary Fiber 9g	1%
Total Sugar 1g	1%
Protein 1g	
Vitamin C 7mcg	17%
Calcium 60mg	1%
Iron 7mg	10%
Potassium 23mg	21%

Ingredient:

- Place 2 tablespoons of olive oil and ¼ cup popcorn in a large saucepan.

- Cover with a lid, and cook the popcorn over a medium flame, ensuring that you are shaking it constantly. Just when you think that it's not working, keep on enduring for another minute or two, and the popping will begin.
- When the popping stops, take off from the heat and place it in a large bowl.
- Add plenty of salt to taste, and if desired, dribble in ¼ cup to ½ cup of melted coconut oil. If you are craving sweet popcorn, add some maple syrup to the coconut oil, about ½ cup, or to taste.

5 Minutes or Less Vegan Snacks

Here's a list of basically 'no-preparation required' vegan snack ideas that you can munch on anytime:

Nutritional Facts

Servings per container	5
Prep Total	10 min
Serving Size	8
Amount per serving Calories	0%
	% Daily Value
Total Fat 20g	190%
Saturated Fat 2g	32%
Trans Fat 1g	2%
Cholesterol	2%

Sodium 70mg	0.2%
Total Carbohydrate 32g	150%
Dietary Fiber 8g	1%
Total Sugar 1g	1%
Protein 3g	
Vitamin C 7mcg	17%
Calcium 210mg	1%
Iron 4mg	10%
Potassium 25mg	20%

Ingredients:

- Trail mix: nuts, dried fruit, and vegan chocolate pieces.
- Fruit pieces with almond butter, peanut butter or vegan chocolate spread
- Frozen vegan cake, muffin, brownie or slice that you made on the weekend
- Vegetable sticks (carrots, celery, and cucumber, etc.) with a Vegan Dip (homemade or store-bought) such as hummus or beetroot dip. (Careful of the store-bought ingredients though).
- Smoothie - throw into the blender anything you can find (within limits!) such as soy milk, coconut milk, rice milk, almond milk, soy yogurt, coconut milk yogurt, cinnamon, spices, sea salt, berries, bananas, cacao powder, vegan chocolate, agave nectar, maple syrup, chia seeds, flax

seeds, nuts, raisins, sultanas... What you put into your smoothie is up to you, and you can throw it all together in less than 5 minutes!

- Crackers with avocado, soy butter, and tomato slices, or hummus spread.

- Pack of chips (don't eat them too often). There are many vegan chip companies that make kale chips, corn chips, potato chips, and vegetable chips, so enjoy a small bowl now and again.

Fresh Fruit

The health benefits of eating fresh fruit daily should not be minimized. So, make sure that you enjoy some in-season fruit as one of your daily vegan snacks.

Nutritional Facts

Servings per container	10
Prep Total	10 min
Serving Size	5/5
Amount per serving Calories	1%
	% Daily Value
Total Fat 24g	2%
Saturated Fat 8g	3%
Trans Fat 4g	2%
Cholesterol	2%
Sodium 10mg	22%
Total Carbohydrate 7g	54%
Dietary Fiber 4g	1%

Total Sugar 1g	1%
Protein 1g	24
Vitamin C 2mcg	17%
Calcium 270mg	15%
Iron 17mg	20%
Potassium 130mg	2%

Ingredients:

- Chop your favorite fruit and make a fast and easy fruit salad, adding some squeezed orange juice to make a nice juicy dressing.
- Serve with some soy or coconut milk yogurt or vegan ice-cream if desired, and top with some tasty walnuts or toasted slivered almonds to make it a sustaining snack.

Vegan Cake

If you are tired or very busy during the week, I recommend you set aside a few hours on the weekends to do your baking. Bake one or two yummy vegan snack recipes to last you the week and freeze them in portions. Find some easy (or gourmet if you wish) vegan cake recipes, muffin recipes, brownie recipes or slice recipes that look delicious, and that you know will satisfy your snack cravings during the week.

Vegan Health Slice

Once again, if you bake it on the weekends, you will not have to prepare your morning and afternoon tea during the week. There are so many delicious recipes nowadays for vegan health slices. There's an apple-crumble slice, oat and nut slice, dried-fruit slice, blueberry slice, chocolate-brownie slice, and so many more delicious recipes! Why not bake a different vegan slice every weekend? This will keep your vegan snacks from becoming boring.

As you can see, your vegan snacks can be very fast and easy to prepare. And it's always a very good habit to get into to do your vegan baking on the weekend so that your mid-week snacks can be hassle-free!

Spicy Apple Crisp

Nutritional Facts

Servings per container	5
Prep Total	10 min
Serving Size	7
Amount per serving Calories	0.2%
	% Daily Value
Total Fat 8g	22%
Saturated Fat 1g	51%
Trans Fat 0g	2%
Cholesterol	2%
Sodium 20mg	0.2%
Total Carbohydrate 70g	540%
Dietary Fiber 3g	1%
Total Sugar 6g	1%
Protein 6g	24

Vitamin C 4mcg	170%
Calcium 160mg	12%
Iron 2mg	210%
Potassium 30mg	21%

Ingredients:

- 8 cooking apples
- 4 oz. or 150 g flour
- 7 oz. or 350 g brown sugar
- 5 oz. or 175 g vegan butter
- ¼ tablespoon ground cinnamon
- ¼ tablespoon ground nutmeg
- Zest of one lemon
- 1 tablespoon fresh lemon juice

Instructions:

- Peel, quarter and core cooking apples.
- Cut apple quarters into thin slices and place them in a bowl.
- Blend nutmeg and cinnamon then sprinkle over apples.
- Sprinkle with lemon rind.
- Add lemon juice and toss to blend.
- Arrange slices in a large baking dish.
- Make a mixture of sugar, flour and vegan butter in a mixing bowl then put over apples, smoothing it over.
- Place the dish in the oven.
- Bake at 370°F, 190°C or gas mark 5 for 60 minutes, until browned and apples are tender.

Apple Cake

Nutritional Facts

Servings per container	8
Prep Total	10 min
Serving Size	2
Amount per serving	
Calories	0%
	% Daily Value
Total Fat 4g	210%
Saturated Fat 3g	32%
Trans Fat 2g	2%
Cholesterol	8%
Sodium 300mg	0.2%
Total Carbohydrate 20g	50%
Dietary Fiber 1g	1%
Total Sugar 1g	1%
Protein 3g	

Vitamin C 1mcg	18%
Calcium 20mg	1%
Iron 8mg	12%
Potassium 70mg	21%

Ingredients:

- 2 oz. or 50 g flour
- 3 tablespoon baking powder
- ½ tablespoon of salt
- 2 tablespoon vegan shortening
- ¼ pint or 125 ml unsweetened soya milk
- 4 or 5 apples
- 4 oz. or 110 g sugar
- 1 tablespoon cinnamon

Instructions:

- Sift together flour, baking powder, and salt.
- Add shortening and rub in very lightly.
- Add milk slowly to make soft dough and mix.
- Place on floured board and roll out ½ inch or 1 cm thick.
- Put into shallow greased pan.
- Wash, pare, core and cut apples into sections; press them into the dough.
- Sprinkle with sugar and dust with cinnamon.
- Bake at 375°F, 190°C or gas mark 5 for 30 minutes or until apples are tender and brown.
- Serve with soya cream.

Apple Charlotte

Nutritional Facts

Servings per container	5
Prep Total	10 min
Serving Size	4
Amount per serving Calories	60%
	% Daily Value
Total Fat 1g	200%
Saturated Fat 20g	3%
Trans Fat 14g	2%
Cholesterol	2%
Sodium 210mg	2%
Total Carbohydrate 7g	210%
Dietary Fiber 1g	9%
Total Sugar 21g	8%
Protein 4g	

Vitamin C 4mcg	22%
Calcium 30mg	17%
Iron 8mg	110%
Potassium 12mg	2%

Ingredients:

- 2 lbs. or 900 g good cooking apples
- 4 oz. or 50 g almonds (chopped)
- 2 oz. or 50 g currants and sultanas mixed
- 1 stick cinnamon (about 3 inches or 7 cm long)
- Juice of ½ a lemon
- Whole bread (cut very thinly) spread
- Sugar to taste.

Instructions:

- Pare, core, and cut up the apples.
- Stew the apples with a teacupful of water and the cinnamon, until the apples have become a pulp.
- Remove the cinnamon, and add sugar, lemon juice, the almonds, and the currants and sultanas (previously picked, washed, and dried).
- Mix all well and allow the mixture to cool.
- Grease a pie-dish and line it with thin slices of bread and butter,
- Then place on it a layer of apple mixture, repeat the layers, finishing with slices of bread and vegan butter.
- Bake at 375°F, 190°C or gas mark 5 for 45 minutes.

Vegan Brownie

Nutritional Facts

Servings per container	3
Prep Total	10 min
Serving Size	7
Amount per serving Calories	20%
	% Daily Value
Total Fat 3g	22%
Saturated Fat 22g	8%
Trans Fat 17g	21%
Cholesterol	20%
Sodium 120mg	70%
Total Carbohydrate 30g	57%
Dietary Fiber 4g	8%
Total Sugar 10g	8%
Protein 6g	

Vitamin C 1mcg	1%
Calcium 20mg	31%
Iron 2mg	12%
Potassium 140mg	92%

Ingredients:

- 1/2 cup non-dairy butter melted
- 5 tablespoons cocoa
- 1 cup granulated sugar
- 3 teaspoons Ener-G egg replacer
- 1/4 cup water
- 1 teaspoon vanilla
- 3/4 cup flour
- 1 teaspoon baking powder
- 1/2 teaspoon salt
- 1/2 cup walnuts (optional)

Instructions:

- Heat oven to 350°. Prepare an 8" x 8" baking pan with butter or canola oil.
- Combine butter, cocoa, and sugar in a large bowl.
- Mix the egg replacer and water in a blender until frothy.
- Add to the butter mixture with vanilla. Add the flour, baking powder, and salt, and mix thoroughly.
- Add the walnuts if desired. Pour the batter into the pan and spread evenly.

Bake for 40 to 45 minutes, or until a toothpick inserted comes out clean.

FINAL WORDS

Thank you for reading this book! This is the 5th book I've written since 2016.

It took me years to write this one, partly because I am a full-time mom and nutritionist. The main reason, however, is that I decided to challenge myself even more this time.

My goal for this guide was to put very complex and technical concepts in the simplest way, so as to make it readable for everyone.

To do what I mentioned above, I accurately selected what I believe are the most useful and effective pieces of advice for you. In my 30 years+ of professional experience I've had the amazing chance to deal with thousands of people of all ages, gender, and personality, and it inevitably has some reflections on my writings.

I don't like to call myself an author, yet I have to admit that I learned a lot while writing books over the past few years. In fact, what I got from those past publications was validation from readers who enjoyed my work and encouraged me to keep writing.

I always value the opinion of readers and take into account criticism as well.

I do believe that reviews are a great way to give someone credit for the work done and I love reading them all the time.

Other readers will do the same before purchasing my books; that's why I give special importance to reviews and I feel bad when getting a bad one.

Anyway, I hope you keep in mind that I am a self-published author, without the huge possibilities that publishing houses have (such as proofreading, special formatting and so on...). However, I hope I accomplished at least the goal I had in my mind - which was to provide you precious information about intermittent fasting, based on scientific studies as well as my own experience, and, most importantly, I hope you learned something new and will act on it to change your life.

Special thanks go to my family, in particular to my beloved husband and my two little daughters, who read this book before than anyone else. I got great feedbacks from them and I am elated about that, even though I think theirs are a little bit biased. After all, they saw me when at nights, often after exhausting workdays, I locked myself up in the study room writing and organizing this guide in the best possible way.

I hope you will keep that in mind too and consider using some seconds of your precious time to leave a review on this book.

I will be GRATEFUL for each one of you.

P.S. I'm a nutritionist, I am a mom, I am a woman but above all... I am a human being. An immaculate work is far from possible, especially when you are alone. So, please, if you wish to report any typos or inaccuracies you encountered in this guide, please consider emailing me at teresamoorenutritionist@gmail.com. I will do my best to answer you and make the requested adjustments.

21-DAYS INTERMITTENT FASTING JOURNAL

MY IF **PLAN**

FASTING PROTOCOL _____

EATING WINDOW _____

DAY(s) I WILL FAST (1) (2) (3) (4) (5) (6) (7)
(8) (9) (10) (11) (12) (13) (14)
(15) (16) (17) (18) (19) (20) (21)

" IT IS BETTER TO TAKE SMALL STEPS IN THE RIGHT DIRECTION
THAN TO MAKE A GREAT LEAP FORWARD ONLY
TO STUMBLE BACKWARD. "

GOALS

_____ ○
_____ ○
_____ ○
_____ ○

MOTIVATION

STARTING WEIGHT	GOAL WEIGHT
_____	_____

21 DAYS INTERMITTENT FASTING JOURNAL

day 01

SHOPPING LIST

○
○
○
○
○
○
○
○
○

NOTES

TODAY I'M GRATEFUL FOR

"

"

TO-DO LIST

○
○
○
○
○
○

EATING WINDOW

(clock: 12 1 2 3 4 5 6 7 8 9 10 11)

21 DAYS INTERMITTENT FASTING JOURNAL

day 02

SHOPPING LIST

- ○
- ○
- ○
- ○
- ○
- ○
- ○
- ○
- ○

NOTES

TODAY I'M GRATEFUL FOR

"

"

TO-DO LIST

- ○
- ○
- ○
- ○
- ○
- ○

EATING WINDOW

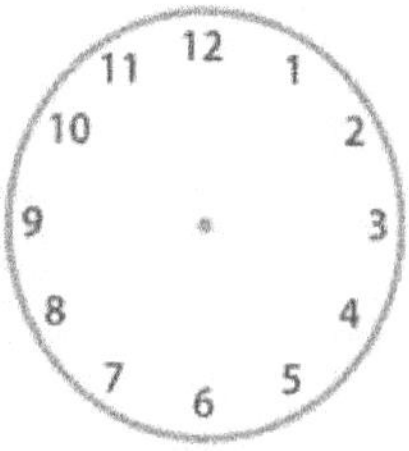

Clock face showing numbers 1 through 12.

21 DAYS INTERMITTENT FASTING JOURNAL

day 03

SHOPPING LIST

○
○
○
○
○
○
○
○
○

NOTES

TODAY I'M GRATEFUL FOR

"

"

TO-DO LIST

○
○
○
○
○
○

EATING WINDOW

day 04

SHOPPING LIST

- ○
- ○
- ○
- ○
- ○
- ○
- ○
- ○
- ○
- ○

NOTES

TODAY I'M GRATEFUL FOR

"

"

TO-DO LIST

- ○
- ○
- ○
- ○
- ○
- ○

EATING WINDOW

11 12 1
10   2
9   *   3
8   4
7   6   5

21 DAYS INTERMITTENT FASTING JOURNAL

day 05

SHOPPING LIST

○
○
○
○
○
○
○
○
○

NOTES

TODAY I'M GRATEFUL FOR

"

"

TO-DO LIST

○
○
○
○
○
○

EATING WINDOW

21 DAYS INTERMITTENT FASTING JOURNAL

day 06

SHOPPING LIST

- ○
- ○
- ○
- ○
- ○
- ○
- ○
- ○
- ○

NOTES

TODAY I'M GRATEFUL FOR

TO-DO LIST

- ○
- ○
- ○
- ○
- ○
- ○

EATING WINDOW

21 DAYS INTERMITTENT FASTING JOURNAL

day 07

SHOPPING LIST

- ○
- ○
- ○
- ○
- ○
- ○
- ○
- ○
- ○

NOTES

TODAY I'M GRATEFUL FOR

"

"

TO-DO LIST

- ○
- ○
- ○
- ○
- ○
- ○

EATING WINDOW

21 DAYS INTERMITTENT FASTING JOURNAL

day 08

SHOPPING LIST

- ○
- ○
- ○
- ○
- ○
- ○
- ○
- ○
- ○

NOTES

TODAY I'M GRATEFUL FOR

"

"

TO-DO LIST

- ○
- ○
- ○
- ○
- ○
- ○

EATING WINDOW

21 DAYS INTERMITTENT FASTING JOURNAL

day 09

SHOPPING LIST

- ◯
- ◯
- ◯
- ◯
- ◯
- ◯
- ◯
- ◯
- ◯

NOTES

TODAY I'M GRATEFUL FOR

TO-DO LIST

- ◯
- ◯
- ◯
- ◯
- ◯
- ◯

EATING WINDOW

21 DAYS INTERMITTENT FASTING JOURNAL

day 10

SHOPPING LIST

- ○
- ○
- ○
- ○
- ○
- ○
- ○
- ○
- ○

NOTES

TODAY I'M GRATEFUL FOR

TO-DO LIST

- ○
- ○
- ○
- ○
- ○
- ○

EATING WINDOW

21 DAYS INTERMITTENT FASTING JOURNAL

day 11

SHOPPING LIST

- ○
- ○
- ○
- ○
- ○
- ○
- ○
- ○
- ○

NOTES

TODAY I'M GRATEFUL FOR

"

"

TO-DO LIST

- ○
- ○
- ○
- ○
- ○
- ○

EATING WINDOW

11 12 1
10 2
9 3
8 4
7 6 5

day 12

SHOPPING LIST

- ○
- ○
- ○
- ○
- ○
- ○
- ○
- ○
- ○

NOTES

TODAY I'M GRATEFUL FOR

"

"

TO-DO LIST

- ○
- ○
- ○
- ○
- ○
- ○

EATING WINDOW

21 DAYS INTERMITTENT FASTING JOURNAL

day 13

SHOPPING LIST

○
○
○
○
○
○
○
○
○

NOTES

TODAY I'M GRATEFUL FOR

"

"

TO-DO LIST

○
○
○
○
○
○

EATING WINDOW

21 DAYS INTERMITTENT FASTING JOURNAL

day 14

SHOPPING LIST

- ○ _____
- ○ _____
- ○ _____
- ○ _____
- ○ _____
- ○ _____
- ○ _____
- ○ _____
- ○ _____

NOTES

_____
_____
_____
_____
_____
_____
_____
_____
_____

TODAY I'M GRATEFUL FOR

" _____
_____
_____ "

TO-DO LIST

- ○ _____
- ○ _____
- ○ _____
- ○ _____
- ○ _____
- ○ _____

EATING WINDOW

21 DAYS INTERMITTENT FASTING JOURNAL

day 15

SHOPPING LIST

- ○
- ○
- ○
- ○
- ○
- ○
- ○
- ○
- ○

NOTES

TODAY I'M GRATEFUL FOR

"

"

TO-DO LIST

- ○
- ○
- ○
- ○
- ○
- ○

EATING WINDOW

21 DAYS INTERMITTENT FASTING JOURNAL

day 16

SHOPPING LIST

- ○
- ○
- ○
- ○
- ○
- ○
- ○
- ○
- ○

NOTES

TODAY I'M GRATEFUL FOR

TO-DO LIST

- ○
- ○
- ○
- ○
- ○
- ○

EATING WINDOW

11 12 1
10   2
9   *   3
8   4
7 6 5

21 DAYS INTERMITTENT FASTING JOURNAL

day 17

SHOPPING LIST

- ○
- ○
- ○
- ○
- ○
- ○
- ○
- ○
- ○

NOTES

TODAY I'M GRATEFUL FOR

"

"

TO-DO LIST

- ○
- ○
- ○
- ○
- ○
- ○

EATING WINDOW

day 18

SHOPPING LIST

- ○
- ○
- ○
- ○
- ○
- ○
- ○
- ○
- ○

NOTES

TODAY I'M GRATEFUL FOR

"

"

TO-DO LIST

- ○
- ○
- ○
- ○
- ○
- ○

EATING WINDOW

11 12 1
10   2
9   3
8   4
7 6 5

day 19

SHOPPING LIST

- ○
- ○
- ○
- ○
- ○
- ○
- ○
- ○
- ○

NOTES

TODAY I'M GRATEFUL FOR

"

"

TO-DO LIST

- ○
- ○
- ○
- ○
- ○
- ○

EATING WINDOW

day 20

SHOPPING LIST

- ○
- ○
- ○
- ○
- ○
- ○
- ○
- ○
- ○

NOTES

TODAY I'M GRATEFUL FOR

"

"

TO-DO LIST

- ○
- ○
- ○
- ○
- ○
- ○

EATING WINDOW

21 DAYS INTERMITTENT FASTING JOURNAL

day 21

SHOPPING LIST

○
○
○
○
○
○
○
○
○

NOTES

TODAY I'M GRATEFUL FOR

"

"

TO-DO LIST

○
○
○
○
○
○
○

EATING WINDOW

PROGRESS CHART

	DATE	WEIGHT	L/R ARMS	L/R LEGS	CHEST	WAIST	HIP
DAY 1							
DAY 2							
DAY 3							
DAY 4							
DAY 5							
DAY 6							
DAY 7							
DAY 8							
DAY 9							
DAY 10							
DAY 11							
DAY 12							
DAY 13							
DAY 14							
DAY 15							
DAY 16							
DAY 17							
DAY 18							
DAY 19							
DAY 20							
DAY 21							

CPSIA information can be obtained
at www.ICGtesting.com
Printed in the USA
LVHW040057121220
673919LV00006B/299

9 781801 323376